Dr. Cohen's

New Hippocratic Diet

Guide

How to Really Lose Weight and Beat the Obesity Epidemic

Irving A. Cohen, M.D., M.P.H.

www.HippocraticDiet.com

Center for Health Information
Topeka, Kansas
www.centerforhealthinformation.com

Copyright 2008 by Irving A. Cohen, M.D.,M.P.H.

Published by
Center for Health Information, Inc.
Suite 22F, 1919 SW 10th Avenue
Topeka, KS 66604
Phone (888) 933-9833
FAX (866) 516-1321

Printed in the United States of America

Library of Congress Control Number: 2008906640

Cohen, Irving A. 1944-

**Doctor Cohen's New Hippocratic Diet Guide:
How to Really Lose Weight and Beat the Obesity Epidemic**

Includes Annotated Bibliography and Index

ISBN 978-0-9820111-9-5

Editor, Alice Heiserman
Cover Illustrator, Darlene Powell
Printed in the United States of America

This book is
dedicated to
those who have suffered
and to those still suffering
from the tyranny of obesity.

Disclaimers

- The information presented in this book has been obtained from authentic and reliable sources. Although great care has been taken to ensure the accuracy of the information presented, the author and the publisher cannot assume responsibility for the validity of all the materials or the consequences for this use.
- Recipes and food choices discussed in this book are intended for those following this plan. These may or may not be the best choices for others.
- All dieters, whether using this or any other diet, are urged to obtain medical evaluation and support. Nothing in this book should be construed as individual medical advice. The reader should consult his or her own physician for such advice.

Contents

Other Books by Dr. Cohen

Addiction: The High-Low Trap
Health Press
ISBN 0-929173-10-4

Coming Soon

The New Hippocratic Diet™ Cookbook
Center for Health Information

To check availability or order these go to

www.CenterForHealthInformation.com

Acknowledgements

There were many people and circumstances that influenced or helped me along the way to completing this book. Many people may not have realized the contribution they made or the impact of their influence on me. This list will be incomplete, for I am sure that when I finish, others will come to mind.

I would like to begin by thanking my patients. The questions they asked and the experiences they recounted all added to the depth of this book. I learned from both the ones who breezed through as well as those who initially struggled before they caught on. They taught me what to emphasize and how to clarify the messages found in this book.

Next, I would like to thank the staff of the Marian Clinic of Topeka and the Sister Sisters of Charity of Leavenworth for caring about the health of those who could not otherwise afford care. Marilyn Page, the Director of the Marian Clinic, had the insight to recognize that the obesity epidemic was having a tremendous toll on the health of those least able to get care. I would like to acknowledge Michael Burns, RN for his help in initiating that program. Special thanks goes to Mary Stewart, RN, ARNP for her help in keeping that program growing and her continuous dedication to patients and their well being.

Next, I would like to acknowledge the pioneers who

recognized both the causes of the obesity problem and the solutions long ago. The works of Hippocrates and Wilhem Ebstein demonstrate that there is little new under the sun. The work of Hippocrates would have been less accessible without the scholarly work of Émile Littré. I must thank Kirsten Evans, M.D., Ph.D. for verifying my translation of Littré. Such historic medical information would be worthless if it were not preserved and made accessible. The following libraries were of key help in locating and accessing those rare texts:

- Clendenning Library of the History of Medicine at the University of Kansas School of Medicine, Kansas City, Kansas
- National Library of Medicine, History of Medicine Department, Bethesda, Maryland
- Bibliothéque Interuniversitaire de Medécine, Histoire de la Medécine, Paris, France

Support was received from Robert P. Hudson Fellowship in Medical Humanities at the University of Kansas School of Medicine for some of the historic research. Special thanks goes to Christopher Crenner, M.D., PhD., chair of the department of the History and Philosophy of Medicine, for all of his advice, guidance and support in that effort. Less would have been accomplished without assistance from Dawn McInnis, rare book librarian, who was always there with suggestions and help. I also am grateful to earlier assistance received from her predecessor, Kelley Brown. Thanks also to David Wilson, M.D., director of the cardiology training program, for support in getting this message to internists and cardiologists.

Less would have been accomplished without all the teachers and mentors who have crossed my path over many years. There is not space enough to name them all, but two giants stand out. Richard Johns, M.D., former chair of the department of Biomedical Engineering at the Johns Hopkins University School of Medicine, showed me that clinical knowledge and systems approaches to health issues were not separate but complemented and strengthened each other. Wallace Mandell, Ph.D., M.P.H., former chair of the department of Mental Hygiene at the Johns Hopkins University Bloomberg School of Public Health, who has remained my friend and mentor over many years, and has helped me understand the complex relationships that exist between behavior and preventive medicine.

This book would not be a reality without the patient guidance I received from Alice Heiserman, my friend and editor. Thank you for keeping me focused.

Finally, there is my family, who has put up with my focus on this topic for so long. My wife, Lauren, has understood, read, critiqued, tested recipes for many years and stood by me. Words can not express my gratitude for that support.

1

Myths and Half-Truths

Do you believe in the tooth fairy or the Easter bunny? Probably not; yet, you may believe many of the myths and half-truths attempting to explain why you are overweight. Many of these myths are keeping you from successfully losing weight and keeping it off. You are not to blame. Popular media and well intentioned government agencies all have helped to spread information that repeats well-known misinformation. The first step in successfully getting to a healthy and attractive weight is setting aside what you thought you knew about why you are overweight. How many of these wrong diet ideas do you believe?

1. Diets Cannot Work
Myth!

Tell that to my patients. They have lost extraordinary amounts of weight that they had been carrying around for years, despite their many unsuccessful weight loss attempts in the past. Some had already developed the biochemical markers for diabetes or the metabolic syndrome, a precursor to diabetes. Those markers returned to healthier values through their dietary change and weight loss. Their need for medication has been reduced. The most successful also had a lifestyle change. As these dieters became more aware of what had caused their past diet failures, their attitudes about themselves changed. A diet that works both effectively and naturally not only helps people lose weight and regain their health but also helps them to develop more positive feelings about themselves. For some, successful dieting gives them the confidence to now succeed in many other aspects of their lives, as well.

2. Overweight People Lack Willpower
Myth!

Do you believe this about yourself? Many overweight people have a significant self-esteem issue because of this myth. Eating the wrong foods actually changes your body chemistry. An ineffective diet can cause you to be constantly hungry when you are trying to lose weight. Your body is chemically signaling you to eat more and so, you do. You are not weak-willed, you are responding to a bad diet. You did not fail, the bad diet failed you.

3. An Inherited Slow Metabolism Keeps You Overweight
Half-truth!

Yes, genetics does play a role in obesity but much less than most dieters believe. True, some people may have a thyroid disorder, which does slow metabolism but this is easily identified through a simple blood test and corrected through thyroid medication. Both "slow metabolism" and "a genetic curse" are convenient ideas to hang on to when you think that you are doing the right things and yet still gain weight.

Two of the groups that have been most maligned about this supposed genetic obesity are Native Americans and

Americans of African ancestry. Yet, historically both of these groups were once fit and slim. Genetically, they still carry that heritage to be fit and slim. Economic conditions burdened them with unhealthy diets long before the remainder of our nation became obese. Today, people of all heritages are in the same boat. Even nations such as India and China are now experiencing obesity and its related problems as they move toward our industrialized lifestyle.

4. People are Fat Because They Do Not Exercise
Half-truth!

I heartily approve of reasonably increased exercise for any dieter. However, it is wrong to say that people would not be overweight if they exercised more. This is a gross oversimplification. Exercise will build muscle strength, improve body tone, and help your self-esteem. However the amount of exercise needed to accomplish any significant weight loss can be enormous. Exercise may strengthen your weight-control program, but it should never replace diet.

Have you ever been to a gym where an exercise group is being led by a twenty-something young lady in spandex? If you are fifty pounds overweight and find it impossible to follow the exercise routine she is leading, think about how much she would be able to accomplish if she had a fifty-pound backpack strapped on! You are already exercising just by carrying around your extra weight. You are neither lazy nor incompetent because you are worn out by carrying this extra burden during your daily activities.

5. Certain Types of Food Will Burn Off Your Fat
Myth!

There are no magic answers nor are there magic foods! Diets that tell you to eat foods that match your hair color or similarly ridiculous ideas do not work. Everyone wants to believe that there are quick and easy answers. How many diet books do you have on your bookshelf that promised magic? The only way a weight-loss diet can work is by changing your metabolic balance so that you burn up your stored energy. The real magic is learning about the right mix and the amount of food that allows you to eat less without feeling hungry or deprived.

6. Eating Fat Makes You Fat
Myth!

Eating more food than your body needs makes you fat, in whatever form it takes! Your body is programmed to take any extra energy you provide and store it for emergencies and lean times. Ounce for ounce, fat does contain more energy than any other food, but that fact is meaningless. To store fat, your body needs to receive a signal from a high insulin level. A high sugar level drives that insulin level! The quickest way to get fat is to stuff yourself with any form of carbohydrate that will turn into sugar. Farmers and ranchers have known this since ancient times. That is why cattle and poultry are fattened by feeding them grain.

7. Cholesterol is Bad for You.
Half-truth!

It is true that an imbalance of cholesterol is bad for you, but cholesterol is an important and vital necessity. Without cholesterol, your body could not make many hormones that are essential to life. The problem with cholesterol occurs when your body creates too much "bad" LDL cholesterol and too little "good" HDL cholesterol. Simply lowering your total cholesterol number without differentiating between good and bad cholesterol can do more harm than good. The right diet can help you achieve a healthy cholesterol balance.

8. Low-Fat Dieting is Effective and Healthy
Myth!

Two recently completed and very large studies backfired on the proponents of low-fat dieting. In both studies, large groups of women were followed for an extended period of time. **Both studies showed low-fat dieting to be highly ineffective in creating weight loss.** In addition, low fat usually means increased proportions of carbohydrates. These high-carbohydrate diets can lower your good HDL cholesterol and put you at risk for diabetes.

9. All Natural Foods are Healthy
Half-truth!

Yes, **real** natural foods are usually healthier, but government regulators have responded to the food processing industry and distorted the meaning of the word "natural" on a food label. Because of this legal mislabeling, you may

5

mistakenly be purchasing artificial "Frankenstein foods" thinking that they are healthy and natural. Instead, these unnatural foods can keep you addicted to overeating. An effective diet makes you aware of foods that are obesity traps.

10. A Fat-Burning State is Bad for You
Myth!

You **must** put your body into a fat-burning state to lose a substantial amount of fat. An ideal diet keeps your body burning the energy it stored as fat without destroying other tissues. Nature has provided us with the ability to store large amounts of fat as energy to be used in lean seasons.

In industrialized nations, most of us do not have large seasonal variations in our diet nor do we go into hibernation as animals do. Therefore, we may constantly overeat, without ever going in to a steady fat-burning state. This simply results in our just continuing to get bigger. When we store energy in the form of fat, we must switch over to a fat-burning state to get rid of it.

11. Surgery is the Only Answer If You are Very Heavy
Myth!

A growing number of people have lost weight as a result of surgery that radically altered their digestive tract. Why was this necessary? Should half of the industrialized world require surgery to be healthy? Surgery has its drawbacks and once done, you are never the same. The goal of surgery is to modify the way you digest your food. There is another answer. Instead of surgery, consider a plan that teaches you how you can eat less without such modification. A diet that works can save you from surgery.

12. Diet Drugs are the Answer
Half-truth!

Yes, some drugs can help you lose weight. However, there is a high price to pay, with side-effects that may endanger your life. The pharmaceutical companies are spending billions of dollars in research to develop new diet drugs. Drugs that promise miracles generate blockbuster profits for drug companies. Dieters who lose weight by using drugs do not learn how their body can naturally maintain weight. The result is that they may have to continue these drugs for the rest of their lives to maintain their weight loss.

In this guide, I hope to show you a plan that has worked for many. The New Hippocratic Diet™ is a starting point to begin your weight-loss journey. As you progress, you will be learning about changes that will keep you healthy once you reach your weight-loss goal. Although no plan can be a perfect fit for everyone, this plan and this diet are working for many who had been unsuccessful in the past.

Try it.

All you have to regain is your health

and your self-esteem.

2

What Is This Diet About?

- **What is the *New Hippocratic Diet*?** This is a weight-reduction diet based upon maintaining a steady rate of fat-burning. I have developed a method (using a computer model) to predict the fat-burning potential of weight-reduction diets. That model showed that the key factors in maintaining efficient fat-burning are the following:
    - Keeping a balance between the amount of food in your diet versus your total energy needs
    - Keeping the proportions among fat, protein, and carbohydrate in your diet balanced for your weight-reduction needs.

    This computer model allowed me to develop techniques for producing a diet providing an effective method for weight-reduction.
- **Why is this important?** Keeping your body in a steady fat-burning state signals your brain that you are relying on burning stored energy. This state of a high degree of fat-burning reduces your appetite and minimizes your sugar-based food craving.
- **Why is this book a *guide*?** This book is limited to useful information, which was most helpful to my dieting patients. There is just enough background to show you why it works, but the emphasis is on how it works and how to use it.

- **Why is it *Hippocratic*?** After developing my computer model, I compared its predications for an optimum diet to other weight-reduction diets, When I did, I found that two important historic weight-reduction diets relied upon these same principles. One was developed by Wilhelm Ebstein, a respected German physician-scientist of the late nineteenth century. That diet was widely used in its day and was found in American medical texts well into the twentieth century. The other, cited by Dr. Ebstein, was the weight-reduction method of Hippocrates, the father of rational Western medicine. Delving into that 2,400 year old recommendation, I discovered that the forgotten dietary advice of Hippocrates fits well with this twenty-first century computer model.

- **Do other diets emphasize fat-burning?** Yes, many of the carbohydrate-avoidance diets attempt to do this. Two of the most popular recent examples were the diets of Dr. Robert Atkins, during the 1970s and again in the 1990s, as well as Dr. Irwin Stillman's in the 1960s. Both popularized low-carbohydrate diets that intended to reduce appetite by inducing the fat-burning state known as *ketosis.*

  Their diets are very different from this diet. Although they recognized that high carbohydrate consumption cancelled out fat-burning, they felt that increasing protein was important. This ignored a basic issue, since if you eat too much protein, some of it will be turned into carbohydrates for energy. My computer analysis revealed that those diets may or may not produce maximum fat-burning, depending upon the balance between dietary components and your own energy needs. This hit-or-miss approach keeps your system on the edge between your body's natural fat-burning state and a hunger inducing sugar-craving state.

- **How does this diet differ from other popular diets?** Many of the newer diets are aimed at dampening blood-sugar swings, largely by eliminating the worst "glycemic load" carbohydrate offenders. This can be helpful, but at the levels they advocate, your brain will continue to crave sugar as an energy source. This will make it difficult to reduce the amount of food you eat to a point where you continue to lose weight.

- **What about diets emphasizing dietary fats?** These vary in their emphasis and claims. Some advocate attempting to greatly reduce or eliminate dietary fat, a move that may actually increase your appetite. Others recommend little restraint on fatty foods to suppress your appetite while yet others emphasize the replacement of "bad fat" with "good fat."

   The computer model used to develop the *New Hippocratic Diet* showed that, unlike these other diets, you must take quantity and balance into account. There are **no "magical foods"** that will make you lose weight without regard to how much you eat. I provide specific recommendations about healthier fats and recommend minimum and maximum amounts.

- **What about the "obesity epidemic"?** This guide provides information regarding food and diet trends that are causing the obesity-related health problems, which are occurring around the world. Whether you need to diet or not, this guide will teach you which dietary trends are pitfalls you should avoid to protect yourself and those around you.

- **What background do I have to provide this information?** Following medical school, I focused my career on the prevention of disease. I received a Master of

Public Health degree from the Johns Hopkins University while I did my post-graduate medical training, completing the Preventive Medicine residency at the Johns Hopkins University. I then went on to become the Chief Resident of Preventive Medicine at Johns Hopkins, supervising other physicians in the largest non-governmental preventive medicine program in the nation.

I am Board-Certified by the American Board of Preventive Medicine in the specialty of General Preventive Medicine and Public Health and I am a Fellow of The American College of Preventive Medicine.

I direct weight-loss programs at two clinics in Kansas, one of my own and the other as a volunteer at a charitable Catholic clinic. I am also an Adjunct Associate Professor in the History of Medicine at the University of Kansas School of Medicine. Recently, I have made presentations concerning obesity and weight-loss at national and international scientific meetings of the following organizations:

- The American College of Preventive Medicine
- The North American Association for the Study of Obesity
- The American Association for the History of Medicine
- The Indian Health Service of the U.S. Department of the Interior
- **What is preventive medicine?** *Preventive medicine focuses on early interventions and changes to protect your health <u>before</u> serious consequences occur.* Unfortunately, the term *"preventive medicine"* is often misused by purveyors of supposedly "magical cures." The true specialty of preventive medicine is one of the recognized branches of

medicine in which physicians may train and qualify. Because our health care system rewards practitioners *after* people become ill, there is a serious shortage of doctors willing to undergo the four extra years of training to qualify in this specialty.

- **Is this the right diet for you?** Perhaps, but you are the one in the best position to answer this. Even if it is not, the information in this guide may still help you understand the problem. I have developed a few questions for my patients that may help you decide if this diet is for you.

    1. *Are you at least eighteen years old?* The guidelines in this book are intended for adults. Children and younger teens may have special nutritional needs. If you intend to use this diet for a younger person, review that decision with a qualified pediatrician or family practitioner before starting.

    2. *Do you need to lose twenty or more pounds?* This diet is not intended for people who would like to lose only a few pounds. Although you may learn quite a bit from reading this book, you will find that this is a diet designed for significant changes.

    3. *Are you pregnant or planning to be soon ?* Do not try to lose weight while you are pregnant. Although some animal species carry their young while fasting, people should not. Your developing baby has many nutritional needs and might miss out on some important substances if you diet while pregnant. Instead, if you are pregnant now, work with your obstetrician regarding weight control during pregnancy. Read the book, but do not start until after you have delivered your baby. If you

want to become pregnant, diet first. Carrying a baby when you have reached a healthy weight will be much safer for both you and your child.

4. ***Are you able to read, write, and understand?*** Since you are reading this book, that answers part of this question, but this diet requires work. I am going to ask you to learn about the foods that you buy and prepare. If you are not sure, you may want to read ahead, *before* you make that commitment.

5. ***Do you prepare your own meals?*** This is not a diet for someone who eats out every meal. If a spouse, companion, or parent prepares your food, ask if are they willing to assist you in your weight-loss. If not, are you willing to prepare your own food?

6. ***Are you medically and psychiatrically stable enough to diet?*** Dieting can bring about significant changes, which are usually for the better. However, if you have any condition which requires close monitoring, consider this decision carefully with your personal physician. This is especially true if you take any medication that requires monitoring through blood tests. If you are currently taking any medication to lower your blood sugar, do not try any form of dieting without close monitoring and medication adjustments by your physician. If you have ever been diagnosed with either an eating disorder or bipolar disorder, avoid dieting unless you are working <u>closely</u> with your physician.

If you do not have any problems with any of these issues, you should be able to diet safely, whether with this or any other diet. Of course, there are always exceptions, so check with a physician, if you have doubts. If you passed these "tests," I have a few more questions you should try to answer to help you decide if you are ready to begin dieting. These are as follows:

Are You Ready to Begin Dieting?

1. *Do you have health problems from your weight?*
2. *Have you tried other approaches and failed?*
3. *Have you successfully lost weight but regained it?*
4. *Are you tired of being overweight?*
5. *Have you ever considered weight-reduction surgery?*
6. *Are you ready for a change?*

If you answered yes to any one of these last six questions, you are definitely ready!

The next chapter should help you understand why we are now facing an obesity epidemic. You need to understand this so that you know that you did not fail in your previous diet attempts.

It is likely that your diet failed you.

3

Why We Are Overweight

The current obesity epidemic is an absurdity. Until recently, the world envied Americans. Statistically, we were taller, thinner, stronger and had an excellent life expectancy. How did we fall so far, so fast? Why are we turning into a nation of shorter, fatter diabetic people with a decreased life span?

Learning the answers to these questions is your key to understanding how choices in your day-to-day activities and food choices influence both your weight and your health. You may think that you know many of these answers already, but, if you do, why are you having a weight problem? We will go beyond the shallow and ineffective answers we hear repeatedly in the media.

The obesity problem in America has not occurred because of automobiles, television, or computers. These are usually blamed and yes, they do contribute to the problem, but the real villain is the manipulation of our food supply on an unprecedented scale. There are several forces behind this. In the 1970s a well meaning but non-medical federal government bureaucracy developed health objectives, which continue to this day. They set important goals encouraging a reduction in dietary fat and an increase in carbohydrates for all Americans. This was the take-off point of the low-fat fad. Government committees responsible for funding the work of university researchers caused scientific dogma to fall into line. Only in the past few years have scientists spoken out strongly, saying these low-fat and high-carbohydrate diets are wrong.

This is a modern version of the fable, *The Emperor's New Clothes*. In that fable, no one wished to be the first to speak out and tell the Emperor that he had been made a fool of. Similarly, scientists who had gone along with our government's edicts about diet were reluctant to point out the problem and appeared to be waiting for someone else to speak out first.

This government-inspired low-fat fad provided a tremendous profit opportunity for the food processing industry. Food processing companies had been creating *faux* or fake foods for years but had to disclose that these foods were imitation. Most consumers looked at these products as second-rate. It costs a lot less to create a fake food than the real product. Now, with the government's blessing, the food industry began to churn out many new versions of these imitation foods coupled with claims that they were healthier! The box on the next page compares what you once got when you asked for cream for your coffee and what the restaurant may give you today. You judge for yourself which product is healthier.

Real Cream   _versus_   **_"Creamer"_**

Ingredient: Ingredients:

1. Cream

1. Water
2. Partially hydrogenated soybean oil
3. Corn syrup solids
4. Sodium caseinate
5. Dipotassium phosphate
6. Sugar
7. Mono and digylcerides
8. Sodium steardyl
9. Lactylate
10. Soy lecithin
11. Artificial colors
12. Artificial flavors

Most Americans today have been so inundated by the combination of advertising claims and well-intentioned advice that they no longer know what to believe. In a society where we are taught to take personal responsibility for our actions, overweight people end up blaming themselves. We find ourselves struggling to lose weight, swimming upstream against a current of unhealthy food choices.

> ## Coincidence?
>
> *Many people do not realize that our food processing industry is controlled by the cigarette industry. It began several decades ago, as these large companies realized that in the future, fewer people would be smoking addictive cigarettes. Searching for an industry that would be shielded from change, the largest tobacco companies settled on the food processors. Many large food processing companies, including trusted old, established brands, became subsidiaries of big tobacco.*

Ingredients in familiar foods changed. Meals that might not have been fattening before now added on pounds. As people began to get heavier, these same food processors came up with new products to appeal to those who want to slim down. These new, more costly "diet" foods often have just the opposite effect, making you hungrier and causing you to eat more. An intelligent but overweight man sat in my office recently and explained how he had been unable to lose weight. He had tried dieting for years and followed the directions for a particular product. Unfortunately, when he ate this prepared dinner, he was so hungry that he had to have two.

It might be funny, were it not so tragic. Unfortunately, there is nothing funny about the consequences of being overweight. We are not alone in the world. About two out of every three adults in America are now overweight but the World

Health Organization sees the same problem emerging in the rest of the world. Even in countries traditionally plagued by malnutrition, this modern horror is showing its face. India and China, as they become industrialized, see the same issues. It is ironic that in those places malnutrition and starvation exist side-by-side with obesity.

Why do you want to lose weight?

- *Health?*
- *Self-esteem?*
- *Appearance?*
    or
- *All three?*

The reality that being overweight creates many health problems has been recognized since the time of Hippocrates, 2,400 years ago. Today, with a national weight problem greater than any other nation, the United States faces the highest health care costs in the world. You may not be interested in solving the health problems of our land, but if enough people, just like you, find that they can slim down naturally, it will help. Do it for yourself and you will be setting an example for your family and those around you. Being overweight is not the sole cause of all health problems, but it is a major factor in many, including those in the list on the next page.

Problems Often Caused by Overweight

• Sudden death	• Fatigue
• Early death	• Depression
• Heart disease	• Sexual problems
• High blood pressure	• Skin problems
• Stroke	• Snoring
• Metabolic syndrome	• Sleep apnea
• Diabetes	• Gastro-esophageal reflux
• Kidney disease	• Asthma
• Arthritis	• and many more

This does not answer the question, why are our foods causing us to be fat? The answer is simple. Ask any child in the third grade and they can tell you that if you eat too much, you will get fat. Ask any farmer or rancher how they fatten animals and they will tell you they stuff them with carbohydrates from grain. Japanese Sumo wrestlers were not born fat. Instead, their trainers stuff them with rice carbohydrates to build up fat and *chankonabe* stew for protein to build muscle to move their fatty bulk around. Artificial foods are loaded with both high levels of carbohydrates and appetite-stimulating flavor enhancers to cover the bland tastes of substitute ingredients. Low-fat substitute foods are often very high in sugar.

This creates very high carbohydrate diets, which are known to be the best way to *gain* weight, not to lose it. Hippocrates taught the ancient world that lesson 2,400 years ago. Farmers and ranchers, both ancient and modern, have always known it. Yet, the Washington bureaucracy spent a quarter-century pushing these fattening diets on the public. All this happened to the delight and profit of the food processing industry and, to some extent, the pharmaceutical industry. The next chapter will explain how this caused you to add pounds and how to reverse the weight problems that it has caused for you.

4

How Food Changed You

Why did these faux foods make you fat? Three important factors were at work:

- **Content**
- **Appetite stimulants**
- **Portion size**

The switch from naturally balanced food products to low-fat carbohydrate rich foods is the number one villain in this story. Most people know that *insulin* has a role in controlling your blood sugar, but not everyone knows about *glucagon*, insulin's balancing companion. These two important hormones work together in controlling your energy balance.

Table 4.1	
Insulin	**Glucagon**
• Increases when sugar in blood is high	• Increases when sugar in blood is low
• Signals body to use sugar	• Signals body that energy is needed
• Signals body to store energy	• Signals body to release stored energy
• Signals body that excess sugar is to be stored as fat	• Signals body to convert fat to ketones

Both insulin and glucagon are produced in your pancreas and have opposite effects. Working as a team, they control the ebb and flow of energy in your body, allowing all of your cells to get the energy they need, whether that energy comes from the food you recently ate or from stored energy, coming from food you ate at an earlier time.

Your body stores its energy in two ways. One way is to create a starch called *glycogen* for short-term energy. Consider it your "between meals" energy source. Another way is to create fat for long-term energy. Consider fat your "off season" energy source. It works fine in nature. Bears eat ravenously during the summer and fall, loading up on carbohydrates which get turned into fat. During their off season, they hibernate and their body switches over to burning their stored fat. People, on the other hand, have gotten very good at storing food supplies for their off season. Today, with most of us shopping at supermarkets, we forget what a short harvest season our ancestors had.

If we eat like bears preparing for winter but never hibernate, we will grow fat. It goes back to that third-grade knowledge. If we eat more than we need, we will get fat. If we want to lose weight, like the bear, we must eat less than we need so our bodies burn up our stored energy.

We wish it were that simple. All we would have to do would be to eat less. That is what people keep telling us, then condemn us as morally weak when we cannot lose. Research scientists can easily demonstrate how almost any diet works, if people behaved like test mice in cages. Unfortunately, that is the extent of the supposed successful testing of many diets.

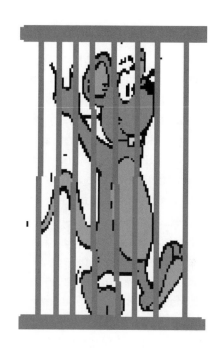

Pay a group of college women to try out a diet in a locked dormitory during a school break and they will lose weight. The true test of a diet should be whether the weight loss holds true once you remove the bars from the cage or the lock from the kitchen.

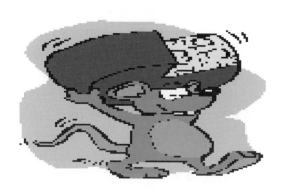

If a diet leaves you constantly hungry, remove the restraints and, like our little mouse, you will want to eat more. If you are very determined, you may lose weight but will probably hate every moment of that diet. An effective diet must do more. A diet that works must get your body to burn fat yet make you feel that you have had enough. Hippocrates described the first such diet and others through the ages have re-discovered the secret. The secret, it turns out, is not a secret at all.

Since your body can only burn two types of energy, everything that you eat gets turned into one of these two fuels. They are sugar, in the form of *glucose*, or fat, turned into a form called *ketones*. Almost every cell in your body can use either one, but like a dual-fueled vehicle or building, adjustments must be made. Cars equipped to run on either gasoline or *E85* ethanol have sensors and computer programs to decide how to adjust the engine based on what fuel mix is running. You, too, have a complex system, with many signal pathways and transmitters, but at the heart of it all is that insulin-glucagon balance.

Initially, our brains always cry out for sugar. When we starve or fast, our muscles switch to burning fat and our body keeps our brain pumped up on sugar. We feel hungry and irritable because we know we are low on energy. That can only last a day or two, because that sugar is coming from our stored up glycogen, our between meals energy supply. After a day or two, as we run very low on sugar, our brains give in and switch to burning fat. Now, we have an ample supply of energy. Although we will be missing other nutrients, we have enough energy for several months. Our hunger is reduced.

In fact, burning fat has other effects. Once we get over the initial discomfort of making the change, we may actually feel better and be able to think more clearly. For some people suffering from a seizure disorder, their brains quiet down and seizures decrease or disappear. A pure fast brings about profound changes in brain chemistry.

Those who knew some things we have forgotten

- *Jesus went to the desert and fasted (for forty days)*
- *Old Testament prophets fasted*
- *Native Americans fasted*
- *Mystics in India fasted*

All experienced a clarity of thought and peace during this religious or mystic experience. Fasting, in many cultures, seems to be a path to inner peace and enlightenment.

Almost a century ago, physicians researched this phenomena and discovered that it was the condition of *ketosis,* the fat-burning state associated with finding ketones in the blood stream, that caused the brain changes that suppressed seizures. With that knowledge, they were able to duplicate the seizure suppression of fasting while allowing patients to still eat. That treatment is still used occasionally today, especially in children who have not been helped by medicines or surgery. Today, it is used infrequently, because it is difficult to follow, requiring a diet of little except fat or oil. In 2008, researchers conducted a large clinical trial proving the validity of that older discovery.

It was this knowledge that allowed me to go one step further, in creating this diet. I found that the mathematical formula developed years ago through research on the therapeutic "ketogenic diet" could be adapted to weight-loss dieting. Ketosis signals fat burning and suppresses hunger, but modern weight-loss diets that stressed ketosis were hit or miss. Most stressed carbohydrate reduction or substituted proteins for carbohydrates and they worked for some but not for others. I know that all too well, because I gained more than fifty unwanted pounds following all the supposed healthy eating recommendations. Those "recommended" diets did nothing for me, which is why I searched for and developed a better way.

On the one hand, eating a diet of almost pure fat would definitely produce ketosis. On the other hand, eating nothing at all would also definitely produce ketosis. I found that the formula developed long ago could be mathematically modified to predict the points in between. The computer model that resulted showed when weight-reduction diets were likely to produce ketosis and when they were not. Diets that are low in calories but just on the edge of ketosis, keep you in constant turmoil. A diet that fails to keep you in fat burning leaves your brain crying out for sugar and you constantly may feel hungry. The computer model demonstrated how all diets could be ketogenic if their total calories were but a tiny fraction of your daily needs.

Diets that were low in their amount of fat but high in carbohydrate quickly stopped being ketogenic as soon as calories increased slightly. Diets that were low in carbohydrate and high in protein could increase calories a little, but they too stopped producing ketosis at some point. This made sense, since the protein you eat gets broken down into amino acids.

Some amino acids get used as replacement building

blocks in your tissues, while the remainder get used as energy. Since energy comes from either sugar or fat, amino acids break down to one or the other. That means that too much protein may produce enough sugar to stop ketosis.

A diet low in carbohydrate, moderate in protein and the balance of its energy coming from fat can stay ketogenic from starvation levels all the way up to fully meeting your daily energy requirements. At the higher energy levels, such a diet would be very high in fat, just like the diet still prescribed for those children having seizures, a regimen that is difficult to follow.

Physicians try to follow the rule *"Primum non nocere,"* meaning **"First, do no harm."** For that reason, I took a conservative approach and have set some additional limits. I set an upper limit for fat at about 70 grams per day, which is about the amount of fat someone who was not losing weight would get from a low-fat diet recommended by heart disease advocates. I set a lower limit for protein of about 40 grams of per day, an adequate amount for most healthy adults. The resultant graph is shown in Figure 4.2 on the next page.

The fat-centered diet line remains high and stays above the dotted line while the other two fall rapidly and lose their fat-burning potential. The filled in area represents what I consider the optimum starting point for most dieters. Although this is what I recommend, I have had people try for less. Once they sense what works for them, people do experiment. My recommendation is conservative and can produce a steady average weight loss of about two pounds (or about one kilo) a week over the long term.

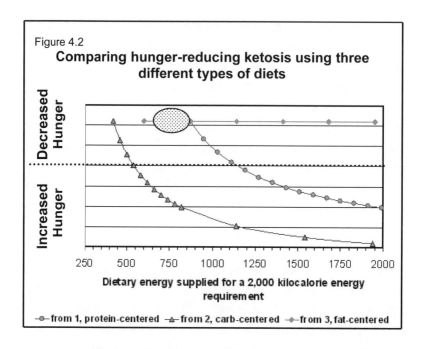

Figure 4.2

Comparing hunger-reducing ketosis using three different types of diets

Those who follow this diet successfully take a few weeks to get the hang of it and understand how their body reacts. Some people will reduce their diet even more, realizing that they can quicken their weight loss. Most patients add exercise, which I heartily recommend. Hippocrates, too, recommended increased exercise, in his *Method of Losing or Gaining Weight.* Exercise helps everyone and you should exercise, <u>to the extent that you are able</u>.

Unfortunately, some diets use the excuse that their diet <u>only</u> works if you exercise. That is a case of a shifting blame to the victim. Let's face it, telling a middle-aged office worker carrying sixty or seventy extra pounds to get into sweats and follow the twenty-something exercise leader at a health club may be futile. Some people will not even go to the gym because they suffer from self-loathing as a result of being overweight and dread being seen in gym clothing. Some brave souls try to keep up, overdoing it and harming themselves.

Try to visualize that spandex-clad instructor carrying the equivalent of your extra weight in a backpack. That is the exercise you are already doing simply going through your daily activities. Do not be shamed into believing you must exercise beyond your means. Instead, start out gradually. For my heaviest dieters, this can mean just walking a little farther each day or going to a "Y" with a pool and joining a water-exercise group. Play a little more with your children, nieces and nephews or grandkids. Be reasonable and work up to the tougher stuff as you lose weight. Let your own body be your guide.

Increasing your activity level through a regular exercise regimen might mean that your loss will be greater than two pounds a week. Either way, be patient. Remember, a loss of two pounds a week, means you can lose a hundred pounds in less than a year.

Have you had enough of charts and graphs? You may be turning pages and asking what the "magic formula" is. Everyone's needs differ, but a good starting point is based on considering a person who needs 2,000 kilocalories of energy each day. This should work well to start for most people but individual adjustment may be needed for some.

The 60-40-10 daily plan	
Fat	*60 grams (but not more than 70)*
Protein	*40 grams (up to 65 if carbohydrates are cut)*
Carbohydrate	*10 grams (or less if you want more protein)*

Think of this **60-40-10** mix as a starting point. If you burn about 2,000 calories each day, this mixture should provide about 37 percent of your energy needs, maintain a moderate to strong state of fat-burning and result in about a two pound weight loss each week. Try to keep your fat consumption up, eating at least 60 grams each day, but try to not go over 70 grams. Special instructions will be given later for those who <u>must</u> restrict their fat intake. Protein should be kept to around 40 grams each day, but may be increased slightly if you decrease your carbohydrate below the 10 grams allowed each day. If you do this, you may substitute 2½ grams of protein for each gram of carbohydrate less than the 10 grams allowed. Although there are minimum "essential" fats and protein needs in anyone's diet, there is no such thing as an essential need for carbohydrates. The carbohydrate allowance can go lower, but you want to include some green leafy vegetables and other foods containing small amounts of carbohydrate each day .

Since these amounts are listed in grams, how do you know what food actually contains? There are several ways to get this information as you select foods. First, using the recipes in this book, you will find estimated counts with each recipe. If you are obtaining recipes from cookbooks or the Internet, look for recipes that include such information. Packaged foods include this information as part of their food labeling. Fresh meat, poultry, seafood and vegetables do not come with product labels, although some markets do provide information sheets. For the rest, use either any standard guidebook that you want to purchase or check the Internet. How to use a nutritional label is explained later in the chapter on shopping. The next chapter suggests how to prepare before starting your diet.

5

Getting Ready

Congratulations! Since you have gotten this far, you are about to try this diet. Take a little time to get ready before starting on this diet. If you have a medical issue which requires monitoring, take the time to meet with your doctor to develop a plan before starting. Otherwise, you are ready to set a goal. Many people start out on a diet without a set goal. It becomes a "Let's see what this can really do." Setting your goal first helps you have direction and purpose. Do not be afraid of doing this, because this diet can really work if you apply it!

Setting your goal realistically is important. If you are reluctant to set a goal because of previous failures, remember that you did not fail before, your diet failed you! The next page provides a body-mass-index (BMI) chart. BMI is important for researchers and statisticians but is not the best way for you to set your personalized goal. You may have been told what "ideal weight" is based on BMI, but that is just a statistical guess based solely on your height.

Rather than BMI alone, use either one of two factors in deciding what your goal should be. Even better, use them together. First, consider your weight history, by asking yourself what you weighed at various points in your life and what you would like to get back to.

Continued on page 38

Finding your BMI Category

Note: BMI treats men and women equally.

	Under-weight	Normal		Overweight		Obese		Extremely Obese
	Less than	From	To	From	To	From	To	More than
BMI	**18.5**	**18.5**	**24.9**	**25**	**29.9**	**30**	**39.9**	**39.9**
Height				Body Weight in pounds				
4' 11"	92	92	123	124	147	148	197	197
5'	95	95	127	128	152	153	203	203
5' 1"	98	98	131	132	157	158	210	210
5' 2"	101	101	135	136	163	164	217	217
5' 3"	105	105	140	141	168	169	224	224
5' 4"	108	108	144	145	173	174	231	231
5' 5"	111	111	149	150	179	180	239	239
5' 6"	115	115	154	155	185	186	246	246
5' 7"	118	118	158	159	190	191	254	254
5' 8"	122	122	163	164	196	197	261	261
5' 9"	125	125	168	169	202	203	269	269
5' 10"	129	129	173	174	208	209	277	277
5' 11"	133	133	178	179	214	215	285	285
6'	137	137	183	184	220	221	293	293
6' 1"	140	140	188	189	226	227	301	301
6' 2"	144	144	193	194	232	233	310	310
6' 3"	148	148	199	200	239	240	318	318
6' 4"	152	152	204	205	245	246	327	327

If you want to know your exact BMI, you can use an Internet calculator provided by The National Institute of Health at http://www.nhlbisupport.com/bmi/bmicalc.htm

Pitfalls using BMI

BMI is a starting point, since it is based on statistics, not on an individual evaluation. It may provide appropriate answers for some but be totally inadequate for others.

Consider a woman who is 5 feet 3 inches tall. Her "healthy" BMI would place her weight between 105 and 140 pounds. Perhaps that is what she weighed when she completed high school, but after raising several children, she now weighs 280 pounds. During that time her bones and muscles remodeled to carry that extra weight. At 280 pounds, she now has 140 pounds of fat, exactly half of her weight. The remaining 140 pounds represents her "lean body mass" and is composed of everything that is not fat.

Her BMI would recommend that she lose at least 140 pounds to be "healthy," but nobody can live without some body fat. BMI has created an impossible goal for her. Most women are healthy when they have about 19 percent to 22 percent of their body weight in fat. Only an extremely fit woman, perhaps a professional athlete, might go a few points lower.

Using a measured body fat percentage, a realistic goal for this woman would be between 173 and 179 pounds. Later, as her body has remodeled at a lower weight, she can be rechecked and a lower goal might then be possible.

Continued from page 35

Next, measure your percentage of body fat to find your healthiest weight. There are many ways to determine that percentage, even if you are doing this by yourself at home.

Measuring your Body Fat at Home

There are two easy ways to measure your body fat in the privacy of your own home. Inexpensive bathroom scales that use electrical impedance to calculate body fat actually work. They are usually accurate to within a few percentage points.

Skin calipers can be purchased for a few dollars through both sporting and medical supply stores. Skin calipers are used to measure the thickness of a pinch of your skin. Professionals measure that thickness at seven spots and use a computer to perform complex calculations. Do-it-yourself calipers, instead, may use a single measure and a simple table to do the same thing. That is close enough for your use, but be sure that your caliper comes with instructions for home use.

Once you estimate how much fat is on your body now, you can determine what your weight should be with a healthy amount of body fat. More information on how to do this is available on-line at *www.HippocraticDiet.com*. A physician, nurse or a well-trained instructor at a local gym can assist you in this. In addition to weight, set other personal goals that you would like to reach. This could be a clothing size, waist measurement, or something personally meaningful.

Next, clean your cupboard and go shopping. If you live alone, get rid of all the foods that made you fat. If you live with others, think about separating some of your food items. Later, your family or companions may want some of the foods you will be preparing, but for now, do not let their preferences influence what you put into your body.

The next pages have two lists of foods, some to clean out and others to stock. Get these basic items to stock for your cupboard, since they are foods that you will use in your diet recipes and meal plan. More information about selecting the right foods is in the chapter on shopping.

When you look at the recommended foods, do not be alarmed if you see foods you do not usually eat. If there are foods to which you are allergic or will not eat for religious or other reasons, just skip them. If you find foods that you have never tried, be daring. This is a great time to break old habits.

In addition to food, there are a few items you will need to test yourself and monitor your weight loss. These are as follows:

- Bathroom scale
- Kitchen diet scale
- Multivitamins with minerals
- Sugar-free fiber supplement
- Ketone test strips
- "Calorie-counting" reference

Each of these items has an important purpose, so do not skip this step. *Continued on Page 42*

Foods to Clear Out

- *Sugar, honey, corn syrup, maple syrup, and other sugary syrups*
- *Flour, corn meal, oatmeal, breakfast cereals and other grain products*
- *Potatoes, rice, peas, beans, spaghetti, noodles, pasta, and other starchy foods*
- *Bread, croutons, crackers, cookies, cakes, muffins, doughnuts, and other baked goods*
- *Soft drinks, except calorie-free products*
- *Alcoholic beverages*
- *Salad dressing containing carbohydrate or MSG*
- *All fruit drinks and sugary fruits.*
- *All soups, unless MSG-free*
- *Desert mixes, unless sugar-free*
- *Processed meats unless MSG-free*
- *Faux foods labeled "low-fat" or "non-fat"*
- *Candy, gum, ice cream treats unless sugar– free or low "net-carb"*
- *Over-the-counter medicines and cough drops containing sugar, if there is a sugar-free alternative*
- *Spice mixes that contain MSG*
- *Worcestershire and soy sauces*
- *Hydrogenated fats, including margarine, shortening, and trans fat*

For now, all of these items will send you back to food cravings. When you get to a maintenance level, you will be able to enjoy <u>some</u> of the items on this list.

Foods to Stock

- *Calorie-free sweetener of your choice*
- *Liquid calorie-free sweetener*
- *Lemon and lime (fresh or juice)*
- *Meats and poultry without added broth*
- *Extra-virgin olive oil*
- *Sesame oil (unrefined)*
- *Fresh or frozen fish (uncoated)*
- *Fresh and frozen green vegetables (but not beans, peas or other legumes)*
- *Celery*
- *Lettuce, salad mixes, and spinach*
- *Avocados and olives (types of non-sugary fruits)*
- *Real heavy whipping cream*
- *Real butter*
- *Real cheese*
- *Real sour cream (not low-fat)*
- *Eggs (high in omega-3 fatty acids preferred)*
- *Nuts*
- *100% pure baking cocoa*
- *Real mayonnaise (olive oil mayonnaise preferred)*
- *MSG-free canned tuna packed in olive oil*
- *Pork rinds (unflavored, MSG-free)*
- *MSG-free sausage and bacon*
- *Sugar-free gelatin (Jello-O™) deserts*
- *MSG-free and sugar-free spice mixtures*

More information on food choice is in the chapter on shopping.

Continued from page 39

The bathroom scale is very important. Many dieters have learned to dread their scale, because of previous frustration with failed diets. Using this diet, you may learn to love your scale, because it helps you track steady progress. Watching your numbers go down can be rewarding.

Although you may already own a scale, see if yours can pass this test. First, can you measure small changes? A useful scale needs to be able to show you changes of half a pound or less. Bathroom scales that have small, unreadable dials or ones that round electronic readings to the nearest pound are not precise enough to be useful here. This diet works best when you get feedback on day-to-day changes. It takes a precise scale to do that. Your scale must also be reliable. Step on and off it a few times. If it gives you the same reading each time, it is reliable. If it does not, toss it in the trash before it does you more harm than good.

Surprisingly, a bathroom scale does not have to be perfectly accurate to work well. If your scale is precise and reliable, it does not matter if it gives you a number slightly different than a more accurate scale in your doctor's office. Just remember to track your weight on the *same* scale and under the same conditions, since you are interested in following the trend that the scale will show you.

You should also test your kitchen diet scale for precision and reliability but it *does* need to be accurate. This will be the tool that lets you judge what size food portions work for you. There are good spring scales but an electronic scale can adjust to allow you to weigh food on a plate, making it easier to use. If you can not find a reasonable scale in a kitchen store, an electronic postage scale from an office supply store works just as well. Find a model with increments of less than an ounce.

A daily multivitamin supplement and mineral is essential for dieters, whether on this or any other diet. Individual needs and food choices will vary, putting dieters at risk of missing some important micronutrient. A daily multivitamin and mineral supplement is your best insurance against that occurring. Although there are claims made to the contrary, for this purpose almost any reliable brand will do.

Daily sugar-free fiber is an absolute necessity on this diet. Your body will process the food found in this diet with very little waste. That will result in little bulk for your bowel movements. Since your intestines have accommodated to larger amounts, the smaller amount of waste may just sit there until gradually, you become constipated. Adding fiber to your diet from the beginning prevents this problem. Do not wait until it happens. There are many fiber supplements at your pharmacy, but be sure they are sugar-free.

The oldest, most reliable supplement is psyllium fiber, in the form of Sugar-Free Metamucil™ powder. It requires you to stir a teaspoon into a glass of water and drink it quickly. Psyllium also comes in a capsule that is simpler to take, but the capsule may not have the same reliability. Some people prefer one of the newer types of tasteless fiber that can be dissolved in your morning coffee or other beverage. Whichever you choose, follow the label directions and adjust the amount to fit your need so that the result is a daily bowel movement without straining or discomfort. The section on reading nutrition labels will tell you more about comparing these.

Ketone test strips may be familiar to anyone who has tried other low-carbohydrate diets. These come in a bottle of fifty and are usually found near diabetic testing supplies in the

Continued on page 45

Dieters and Gallbladder Disease

Your gallbladder is a small storage sac that holds bile produced by your liver. This supply of bile is then dumped into your intestine whenever needed to help break down long strings of fat before they are absorbed. Some people develop stones, inflammation, and even infections in their gallbladder. If your gallbladder has been surgically removed, you still produce bile but it can not be supplied in large quantities when needed.

Unfortunately, the following groups have a statistically higher risk of having gallbladder problems:

- Women, especially those who have had children (the risk goes up with more children)
- People who are over 40
- People who are overweight
- People who are dieting

Keep this in mind when dieting. If you find yourself unable to handle fat, developing symptoms such as fullness, nausea, bloating or diarrhea after eating fat, try changing to a different fat such as MCT oil (explained on page 45) and talk to your doctor about medication.

If you develop abdominal pain, tenderness or discomfort, particularly in your right upper abdominal area under your rib cage, seek medical help promptly.

pharmacy. They are called *Ketostix™* or generically *Ketone Test Strips*. We will discuss how and why to use them shortly.

Many dieters already own a calorie-counting reference book of some sort. Most any one will do, if it shows grams of fat, protein, and carbohydrate for common produce, meats, and fish. Most of these books are thick from detailed and unnecessary listings of packaged products. The same information is always available on the package itself, where it will be up to date. You will need it for the fresh items that are not packaged. You may also be able to find that information on the Internet and skip the book.

This is enough preparation for most people. However, if you are being followed closely by a physician, for any reason, discuss your plan to diet before you begin.

If you have ever had gallbladder disease or have difficulty digesting fat, you should find one extra product called MCT (*for Medium-Chain Triglyceride*) oil. MCT is a form of fat that is digestible without your body first breaking down the long chain of fat molecules that are normally strung together. It allows dietary fat energy to be used even for people who can not easily digest fat. If you suffer from this difficulty, substitute MCT oil for other fats in the recipes found here.

Finding MCT oil may be difficult. Hospital pharmacies carry it, in an expensive pure grade. If a natural food store near you does not stock it in a consumer grade, you may be able to order it online or by phone. If you cannot find MCT oil, you may wish to try using unrefined coconut oil, available at specialty and natural food stores. It is a natural source of medium-chain triglycerides.

In addition, there is a medication that your doctor can prescribe called **ursodiol** *(or ursodeoxycholic acid),* which is prescribed as *Actigall™* and under several other trade-names.

Research has shown it can prevent gallstone formation in many dieters. If you experience problems when eating fatty foods, talk to your doctor about starting this medication <u>before</u> you begin to diet.

Finding MCT oil

*Suppliers and addresses can change,
so check*

www.HippocraticDiet.com

*for suggestions about obtaining MCT oil if
it is not available locally.*

The chapter that follows will guide you through starting your diet by turning on your fat-burning switch.

6

Starting to Diet

This diet has three phases, *starting, fat-burning* and *maintenance.* This chapter is about starting, which is the shortest but hardest part of this diet. Fortunately, there are many people who can start this diet easily, but others may feel tired and irritable for a day or two. I advise my patients to start on a weekend, when they are not working, traveling, or scheduling important events.

The purpose of this starting phase is to rapidly move you off the "dietary cusp." A cusp is a sharp point, in this case at the intersection of sugar-burning and fat-burning. All weight-loss diets should have burning fat as their goal, but most diets keep you right at this intersection. Imagine yourself sitting on a sharp point. Keeping you at this point is very uncomfortable and makes many diets fail. When you are between sugar-burning and fat-burning, you can feel irritable, weak, confused, and you may be obsessing about food. *The starting phase of this diet is designed to get you past that point and into comfortable fat-burning as quickly as possible.*

The simplest way to tell your body to burn fat is through total starvation or fasting. If you eat absolutely no food, your body makes the switch to burn its stored fat in a matter of days, but some people will have a difficult time with a total fast. This starting diet provides alternative strategies for those initial days. These strategies provide a partial fasting alternative and can be easier than observing a total fast.

The quickest strategy is called ***calorie-free partial fasting*** and the second calls for ***fat-centered partial fasting***. Using either one, you deprive your body of sugar. That forces the hormones and neurotransmitters that regulate your hunger to cry out for sugar. Your body is then forced to burn its emergency supply of glycogen, the starch that provides a quick sugar fix. As you burn up that glycogen supply and sugar becomes scarce, your muscles begin burning fat, but your brain resists the change, and keeps using your remaining sugar. Your brain cells will wait while your sugar supply runs low. *Because of this, you may find yourself becoming anxious, grouchy or ill-tempered and have difficulty concentrating.* **Schedule your personal events accordingly.** *If you are an airline pilot or a brain surgeon, take a few days off!*

Once your change-over is complete, you will begin to feel re-energized. When your brain starts burning fat, subtle changes occur in your brain chemistry and neurotransmitter levels. Deliberate fasting has been used to promote inner peace for thousands of years and in many cultures.

Getting High on Fat?

"Mary" attended a reunion after starting her diet. She worried that she would feel out-of-place, by not having alcohol. Instead, she reported that as she circulated, with club soda in hand, she felt wonderful. She said "I think the ketosis kept me mellow, feeling the high I would have felt having a drink, without touching alcohol."

Similar brain-chemistry changes may be the mechanism responsible for the benefits of a diet high in fish oil for mental health issues. This is an important breakthrough now being studied around the world .

Once you have reached this fat-burning state, this diet is intended to keep you there. This is very different than remaining on that uncomfortable edge with other diets.

During this initiation phase, you may lose weight fast. This is sometimes called "water-loss" but is actually the result of glycogen loss. Glycogen weighs more than fat, so you lose weight faster when burning it off. In addition, glycogen is bound to water so the idea of water-loss is partially correct. This rapid loss of a few pounds is very important, but this is not the desired stage of steady fat loss. It is this rapid loss of weight that allows some diets to make claims about losing so many pounds in just a few days.

Exactly how long this transition to fat-burning takes will vary, because some people may have become physically addicted to high-carbohydrate foods. The important enzyme pathways that turn stored fat into burned-up energy may be weak. If skipping a meal puts you in a bad mood or keeps you from thinking clearly, you may have weakened pathways for burning fat. If so, allow yourself a little extra time for this starting phase.

Atrophy

If you have ever had to have an arm or leg in a cast, you may know about atrophy. Your body is designed to "use it or lose it" in many ways. As cells wear out, your body conserves resources by favoring replacement for those things that are the most active. When your cast comes off, your limb may be weak and need special exercises or physical therapy to regain the strength it had before it was inactive.

Similarly, brain connections, neurotransmitter levels and enzyme pathways may respond to use. If you never give your body the chance to burn its fat, you will be trying to turn on switches that could be rusty and stiff. Be patient, your body's abilities will come back.

Your choices for calorie-free partial fasting are simple. During those few days, do not eat anything containing significant amounts of calories. Limit what you eat to the following list:

Things that You Can Have During a Calorie-Free Fast

- Water, coffee, tea and calorie-free diet soft drinks
- Artificial sweeteners
- Sugar-free chewing gum
- Celery
- Most spices (excluding MSG)
- Medicines prescribed by your physician
- Sugar-free vitamin and mineral supplements *(required)*
- Sugar-free fiber supplements *(required)*

You should drink plenty of water or other fluids during this time. Following this method should send your body into fat-burning as rapidly as a total fast, without feeling as deprived.

However, a calorie-free fast may be too severe for some. If you try this and find yourself ready to give up, switch to the plan for a fat-centered partial fast. You can add anything on this next list, provided that you do not exceed sixty to seventy grams of fat each day. Because these may contain small amounts of protein and carbohydrate, this may stretch out your starting phase for another day.

Items on this next list are explained in the sections on recipes and shopping. Read those sections, so that you do not get the wrong product or use a recipe too high in the wrong ingredients.

Foods You Can Add to a
Fat-Centered Partial Fast

- *Extra-virgin olive oil and unrefined sesame oil*
- *Real heavy whipping cream (not prepared whipped cream!)*
- *Real sour cream*
- *Real mayonnaise*
- *Real butter*
- *Real homemade cream soda*
- *Sugar-free Jell-O™ (in limited amounts)*
- *Real homemade whipped cream*

Use the sesame or olive oil, mayonnaise and the bleu cheese dip (found in the recipe section of Chapter 14) on the celery. The homemade real whipped cream (also in the recipes) adds sparkle to your Jell-O.™ Use the cream in your coffee. Follow the recipe for real cream soda. *"Real"* is the key word in several of these. You may have become so accustomed to substitutes that the use of real ingredients instead of sugary counterfeit substitutes may seem strange. Follow the recipes closely until you learn the basics. Later, you are free to go ahead and develop your own variations. Although you will only be on the starting phase of this diet for a few days, continue to enjoy some of these treats throughout your diet.

You only need to stay in this starting phase briefly. Most people will take about two to three days. Once your body starts to naturally break down its stored fat, chemical changes in your blood will signal that you are ready to move on to the fat-burning phase of the diet and resume eating.

How will you know when you reach this stage? A few people may notice some difference in their urine and a fruity taste in their mouths, but the only reliable way to know when fat is coming from storage is a simple home test. You will have completed the starting phase when this test becomes positive.

You will now get to use ketone test strips that you purchased. To use a test strip hold it by the plastic end while dampening the paper end in your urine stream. If you find this awkward, you may catch some urine in a disposable cup and dip the test stick. Either way, it takes just a drop to get it damp. Remove it and wait fifteen seconds, as directed by the instructions that come with it. If you are burning enough stored fat to show in your urine, the indicator will change color. Compare the strip to the comparison chart on the side of the bottle, which resembles the picture below, although your chart will be in color. The colors will vary between a pale beige and a deep reddish-brown brick color.

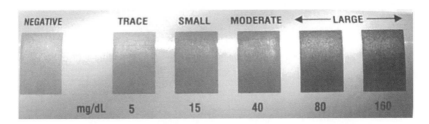

Urine testing is never as accurate as blood testing, but it is painless, inexpensive, and done in the privacy of your home. For the purpose of monitoring your diet, this test is good enough.

Do not expect it to show much on the first day, but by the second, or third day the color should reach *moderate* or *large*. Once you reach that point, you are ready to move on and start following the suggested meal plans and recipes.

7

Eating to Lose

Now that you are in solid fat-burning, it is time to begin eating. You already may have lost a few pounds while you were getting started. Now, you will be able to eat a variety of foods in the right amounts and proportions. This balance should keep you from feeling deprived or hungry while you continue to lose weight at the rate of two or more pounds each week. The daily plan shown here is an example, with full plans and recipes provided in Chapter 14.

Some people prefer to be told exactly what to eat every day, while others prefer independence in their food selections. Consider the meal plans and recipes a starting point. Later, in Chapters 9 and 14, you will see how simple it is to create new recipes or modify others to fit this diet. You may share your creations with others at www.HippocraticDiet.com. Some of the recipes given in Chapter 14 originated with dieters like you.

I have found that most people who are successful like to start out by closely following recipes and meal plans for a few days. Once they see how easy and effective these are, they begin to experiment and change things. Keeping close watch on your own progress is the best way to see what changes really work well.

All the meal plans roughly follow the 60-40-10 plan. These are for a person who uses about 2,000 kilocalories or

---

A Typical Day's Meal Plan

Breakfast
Coffee (or tea or chocolate)
made with real cream and non-calorie sweetener
Large egg, cooked your way
Strip of thick sliced bacon
(or msg-free sausage or fried smoked salmon)

Lunch
Non-calorie beverage
Green salad with extra-virgin olive oil based
dressing

Dinner
Non-calorie beverage
Small portion salmon fried in olive oil (or butter)
with spices
Asparagus dressed in real mayonnaise curry
dressing
Chocolate cream desert

Snack
Portion of nuts

---

more of energy daily. Some people who are smaller, older, or less active may burn fewer calories and need to adjust their meal plan amounts slightly downward.

When you switch from the initiation phase to this phase of your diet, it could not be simpler. You will be pleasantly surprised at how you feel full, eating portions that are much smaller than you were used to in the past. Start by following the meal plans and recipes supplied in this book.

The 60-40-10 daily plan	
Fat	**60 grams** *(but not more than 70)*
Protein	**40 grams** *(or up to 65 if carbohydrates are cut)*
Carbohydrate	**10 grams** *(or less if you want more protein)*

Swap around those things you do or do not like but keep an open mind about recipes and foods you have not tried before. Continue to use the ketone test strips to be sure you stay at a moderate to high level of ketosis. Watch your scale and see if you can detect a quarter pound loss each day. See what works for you and adjust and personalize it to meet your needs.

How do you know what works for you? You will get to personalize your diet by tracking your progress, a skill you will learn later, using Appendix A for tracking your progress. After a few weeks you will get so used to your new diet that it will become second nature, but you should initially keep close track of your diet. The extra effort of jotting down a few notes daily can make the difference between you cruising along on your diet without difficulty or bumping up and down with plateaus and slow progress points.

All diets are infamous for plateaus, periods when the diet appears to not be as effective as when it first started. Many people think that they have reached a biologic "set point," although still overweight. That is another misconception that keeps people overweight.

Earlier, I mentioned the additional exercise workout you have been getting, just by dragging around that extra weight. As you diet, two things occur. One is that you start using energy pathways that are rusty and weak. They may not have gotten much use in years. As you diet, you are exercising those energy pathways and they begin to operate more efficiently. That will change your energy balance, because your body realizes that you are in an energy deficit, and it is squeezing every last drop of energy out of the food you eat and your stored energy. As you lose fat, you are hauling less weight around, causing you to need less energy for the same routine daily activities. This makes you believe you have reached a set point, a weight you cannot go below. No, you have not. If you are still overweight and your energy needs have dropped, adjust your diet. *The 60-40-10 plan is a starting point.* Individualize it to your energy needs as they decrease.

Are You as Smart as Your Car?

Your car has a computer to vary the ignition timing and fuel injection between performance and economy modes. It can detect when you switch the octane level of your gasoline. Your body is infinitely smarter than your car. Right now, if it had your car's computer, it might be running in the trailer-towing mode.

   The sample meal plans exist because people asked for more information when they were starting to diet. Rather than calculate what works for them, they were asking for a simple starting point. Some people continue to use them as a guide, but most dieters pick and choose the recipes and combinations they like after the first few weeks. Even using these starting recipes and meal plans, track them well. They are all approximations and cooking methods, even different brands of products or cuts of meat may alter them. The most useful adjustments to your diet will be those you develop yourself.

Some people were disappointed when I suggested keeping track of their diet because they had been unsuccessful in the past, having kept a food diary at sessions at a weight-loss chain. They had gone to that trouble and still had not been successful losing weight. When they found that they were losing weight on this diet, tracking progress and adjusting their diet for steady loss made the extra effort worthwhile.

Every day of this diet offers new insight into what works and what does not. Food cravings that suddenly return can sabotage either your weight-loss or your maintenance. Many days a dieter brings the label from a suspicious food into our group meetings. More often than not, we find a triggering appetite stimulant cleverly hidden in the ingredients list. You will learn about avoiding those hidden things in the chapter on shopping. It is the one chapter I suggest you re-read periodically. There are so many ways the food companies can sabotage your diet that shopping will become a new experience.

When you complete your partial fast and begin to eat, you will be happy to eat again but skeptical about the small portion sizes. Most of my dieters have been very surprised to learn that they were satisfied with these seemingly small portions. That is the magic of your body. The diet is not magic, but your body is. Despite years of abuse, it can return to knowing what is healthy and what it needs.

Those who are skeptical will try to cheat. They will reason that they can diet more slowly by not trying to create such a major change. They are wrong. Although they may lose a few pounds, they will be fighting constantly. Why? Because the conditions that signal your body to go into maximum fat burning with reduced hunger will be defeated by this cheating behavior. Instead of having an easier time, as they had assumed, they make it much harder. Instead of my lecturing them on their folly, I let the group teach them by example. When they see and hear how other members are rapidly losing weight by not taking shortcuts, they eventually change and the pounds begin to easily slide off for them, too.

Soon, I will explain how to track your progress and determine what works for you. Using the daily plans given here as a general diet is a great starting point for the average person, but who is that? Keeping a close watch on your daily progress and choices will make this plan customized and more effective for you.

You are not helpless in this fight for better health and this is not just a diet, it is a choice to follow a winning lifestyle. As you successfully diet, you will realize that you have regained control over this segment of your life, it can give you the confidence to take control of other, seemingly unrelated, areas of your life. The first choices you will make will be in the supermarket and in your home, as you learn how to fight the obesity epidemic for yourself and your loved ones.

Are you Suspicious?

You may have read about how, in the past, the tobacco company scientists manipulated cigarettes using additives that made their product more addictive.

In August 2005 the *Chicago Tribune* newspaper published a series of investigative articles. They revealed collaboration between tobacco company brain chemistry experts and food scientists working at a popular cookie company, which is owned by the tobacco giant.

Do you wonder what they discussed?

8

Foods to Avoid

Insanity has sometimes been defined as repeating errors of the past and expecting them to come out differently this time around. For you, this means that you must be open to letting go of particular foods that are obesity traps. If you live alone, clean your cupboards. Give away or toss out any of the food discussed in this chapter. Set aside your feelings of what you paid for something. Do not use the excuse that a guest might ask for it.

If you live with others, this is a more complicated task. You may not wish to impose your food choices on others. You are dieting, they are not. However, as they see you are serious about your weight-loss program and they begin to see the results, hopefully, they should be supportive and be willing to compromise.

Start out by cleaning out the most unhealthy foods that no one in your household should be eating. Keep the special foods you obtain for your diet separate from other family foods. Many dieters have learned that once they start cooking with real ingredients, their family wants to share these new dishes, but do not start out forcing your choices on others.

I have repeated a brief list of foods to avoid from the earlier chapter on getting ready to begin. This chapter provides you more information about avoiding foods that may sabotage your weight-loss. Five important food selection rules to follow are the following:

1. **Avoid faux-foods**
2. **Avoid flavor enhancers**
3. **Avoid engineered fats**
4. **Avoid unnecessary carbohydrates**
5. **Read all labels suspiciously**

Avoiding faux-foods

Faux is the French word for fake. If you are buying inexpensive costume jewelry with fake stones, faux is good. In food, it is not. Pseudo-foods, even Frankenstein-foods, are some other terms that can be used to describe the unhealthy substitutes concocted by the food processing chemists. The opposite of faux is real. You may notice that I am avoiding the term "natural" to describe real foods. I do this simply because the food manufacturers have legally kidnapped that word, assigning it a new meaning that you will find hard to believe.

You are probably eating less real food and more faux-food than you imagine. What is the difference? Go to your kitchen cupboard or refrigerator. Read the ingredients list on any food you pick up randomly. Isn't it amazing? The question to ask yourself is "What are these ingredients and what do they do?" It is very likely that you do not know what half of them are or why they belong in this particular food. If that is the case, it is probably a faux-food. Please, do not blame the farmer. Farmers still supply real food but the profit is in the processing.

One example is the substitution of chemicals for real cream in dairy products. Butterfat is the expensive part of the milk. Dairy farmers are paid for their milk based upon the

Continued on page 66

Foods to Clear Out

- *Sugar, honey, corn syrup, maple syrup, and other sugary syrups*
- *Flour, corn meal, oatmeal, breakfast cereals and other grain products*
- *Potatoes, rice, peas, beans, spaghetti, noodles, pasta, and other starchy foods*
- *Bread, croutons, crackers, cookies, cakes, muffins, doughnuts, and other baked goods*
- *Soft drinks, except calorie-free products*
- *Alcoholic beverages*
- *Salad dressing containing carbohydrate or MSG*
- *All fruit drinks and sugary fruits.*
- *All soups, unless MSG-free*
- *Desert mixes, unless sugar-free.*
- *Processed meats unless MSG-free*
- *Faux foods labeled "low-fat" or "non-fat"*
- *Candy, gum, ice cream treats unless sugar–free or low "net-carb"*
- *Over-the-counter medicines and cough drops containing sugar, if there is a sugar-free alternative*
- *Spice mixes that contain MSG*
- *Worcestershire and soy sauces*
- *Hydrogenated fats, including margarine, shortening, and trans fat*

For now, all of these items will send you back to food cravings. When you get to a maintenance level, you will be able to enjoy some of the items on this list.

Continued from page 64

amount of butterfat it contains. The remainder of the cow's milk is much less valuable. If the same amount of butterfat can be used to produce a pint of real sour cream or four pints of faux sour cream, which do you think brings the food processor more money?

The low-fat craze created a tremendous profit generator for food processors. The chemical companies that supply additives to the food processing companies are good at what they do. Good for them, bad for you. To see this difference, look in your supermarket dairy case for real sour cream. The ingredient list will list only one item, *cream.* Nothing needs to be added to a real product to make it taste like the real thing or look like the real thing or feel like the real thing. Now, look at the low-fat or non-fat sour cream sitting right next to it. It lists ingredients to artificially give it flavor, texture, and color. Take away the actual cream and you are left with a chemical soup.

Faux-foods are bad for you for many reasons. Typically, when a real ingredient is removed, unhealthy amounts of sugar are added. Many low-fat foods, which dieters think are lower in calories, often have enough sugar added to have far more calories than the real product. Faux-foods contain a mixture of chemicals designed to fool you by attempting to imitate not only the flavor, but also the texture and color of the real product. The most notorious among these are the glutamate flavor-enhancers, substances that dieters must avoid.

When original, real fats are removed, they are often replaced by the cheapest vegetable oils, deliberately hydrogenated to physically resemble what they replaced and full of dangerous *trans*-fatty acids. Real foods are typically

---

Have You Ever Visited
Colonial Williamsburg, Virginia?

Homes in Colonial Williamsburg are decorated in lovely and unique soft pastel shades, which modern paint companies have tried to duplicate. When the original colonists separated the butterfat from milk, they used that butterfat to produce butter and cheese. They used the leftover product for whitewash or tinted it for paint. Today, dairy processors sell as this product as non-fat skim milk.

---

fresher, while faux foods may have a much longer shelf life than real food. *(Who ever heard of cardboard going stale?)* Achieving that long shelf-life often requires the addition of even more worrisome chemical preservatives.

Sometimes laws and regulations require faux-foods to use truthful names and sometimes they do not. Look for the word ***"Real"*** in the product name but always continue to read the ingredient label. "Real mayonnaise" by regulation, must contain eggs and oil in certain amounts, while other "light" mayonnaise and other imitation spreads do not contain the same amounts of these ingredients. Both real and imitation versions usually contain spices. Although flavor enhancers may exist in either version, they are more likely to be found in the imitation substitute. Similarly, real butter does not need artificial ingredients but margarine is always artificial. Still, you need to be aware that not all butters are the same. Butter usually contains cream and salt, yet some processors add flavor and texture enhancers, so once again, read the ingredient label carefully. With time and practice, you will learn which products are the purest, which brands sold in your region are real food and which are not. It is a sad commentary that it is not always possible to find pure products but try to avoid faux-foods and eat pure foods wherever possible.

I have been using words such as *"pure"* and *"real"* avoiding the use of the word *"natural."* Most people think they know what "natural food" means and may picture a small grocer selling only the purest organically grown products direct from a small local and family-owned farm. Unfortunately, the food-processing industry has stolen that meaning from us. If we go to the dictionary, we can find more than a dozen meanings listed for the word *"natural."* When we think of the word *"natural"* regarding food, we might think of the dictionary definition **"not altered or treated or disguised."** My dictionary even uses *"natural coloring"* as an example of that definition. It would seem common sense to use this definition, and, if so, consumers could have confidence that a natural product was the real thing.

Unfortunately, there is another dictionary definition. The one that the food industry regulators have chosen. That definition is **"present in or produced by nature."** Using that definition, **any product is *"natural"* if it is made from something that ever grew, moved, or crawled**, whether or not it has any relation to the food in question!

I must warn you, this is a true example which may make you nauseous. Products such as strawberry yogurt and strawberry ice cream may contain a red dye listed as "natural coloring." Many consumers would assume that a "natural" coloring for strawberry would come from strawberries. However, in the strange world of legislation and regulation designed by the food-processing industry, this additive is as far from strawberry as you can imagine. The "natural" coloring used is often cochineal dye, a red dye made of the dried and pulverized bodies of female cochineal insects of the beetle family *Dactylopiidae*. The food companies could easily use a red dye made from other chemical substances, but if they did, they would be required to identify it as artificial coloring. Instead, to fool the health conscious consumer who is trying to avoid additives, they use crushed, dried beetle juice!

There is a consumer movement to stop this misleading labeling for this one particular insect product. Recently, the pro-consumer group, Center for Science in the Public Interest (CSPI), petitioned the U.S. Food and Drug Administration to require different labeling for this one particular additive.

Who Can You Trust?

It is tough to avoid faux-foods and unwanted ingredients. I once visited the retail shop of a meat-packing plant in an Amish farm area. I was shocked when I read the list of ingredients for their *"Farm-Fresh Amish Country"* processed meat products because they contained the same preservatives and glutamate flavor-enhancers as any cheap supermarket product. Since then, I have learned that these small producers buy their ingredients pre-mixed and cannot purchase additive-free spice mixtures.

Read every product label carefully !

Unfortunately, even if this occurs, this will not address the larger issue. Changing or restricting the labeling for this particular item, still does nothing to restrict the continued misuse of the word *"natural"* on thousands of other items that are similarly misleading. **Protect yourself from faux-foods by never trusting the word *"natural"* on an ingredient list** without a specific and clearly understandable explanation of what the so-called natural ingredient actually is, where it came from, and why it is present in that food product.

Avoiding Flavor Enhancers.

When I suggest avoiding flavor-enhancers, do not think that flavor-enhancers are some sort of spice. Spices have a taste or a fragrance of their own, which may complement the taste of a food. Flavor enhancers have no inherent taste. Their role is to amplify whatever other flavors may be present, whether those flavors are real or artificial.

MSG, which stands for **monosodium glutamate** is the prototype of all the glutamate flavor enhancers that dieters must avoid. You may have heard about controversy surrounding MSG for years; yet, many of my patients do not even understand why it is added to processed food. Some people wrongly believe that it is a preservative of some sort. It absolutely is not a preservative, but just the opposite. As a powerful flavor-enhancer, it was first used in Asian cooking not to preserve food but to make old, stale food taste fresh and flavorful.

Simply put, MSG works by turning up the volume in our taste buds. In much of Asia, food is never brought to the table with a knife. Instead, it is cut into bite-sized portions before cooking. If this is done too far in advance, the cut food loses its freshness and is less flavorful. Adding MSG makes the stale food taste fresher, by amplifying the flavors that remain.

I am told that MSG and related compounds rarely occur in nature, with the possible exception of these sources:

- Kombu, a Japanese seaweed condiment used as a flavoring.
- Fermented fish sauce, which has been used in some form in the West as a flavor-enhancer since ancient times.
- A rare form of bat found only in one small island of the South Pacific. Islanders consider it quite tasty but it has been suggested that it may be related to an unusual neurological disorder found on that island.

A Japanese chemist named Kikunae Ikeda invented synthetic MSG a century ago. He was curious as to why the seaweed condiment Kombu his wife cooked with always seemed to make her cooking tastier. After identifying the MSG compound, he found a way to synthetically produce it. Ikeda became wealthy, as MSG spread rapidly throughout Asia, largely because of the food freshness problem due to the Asian cooking style. It was eventually added to Japanese canned foods to make them taste fresher.

The rest of the world did not pay attention to MSG until after World War II. Americans returning from Asia had noticed how the Japanese canned products seemed to taste fresher and more flavorful than their American equivalents.

American food processors woke up to this supposed "miracle" of modern chemistry and began to add it to their products. Popular cookbooks advised young housewives to add a teaspoon of MSG to all their dishes. However, by the mid-1960s, warnings about MSG toxicity were beginning to be heard. Consumers became alarmed and MSG became a dirty word. Since then, the food industry has played a cat-and-mouse game with the public. The use of MSG in processed food continues unabated, but it is often disguised in such a way that the consumer is unaware of it.

The efforts of the food-processing industry to cloud the issue are reminiscent of earlier efforts when the tobacco industry was trying to pretend that tobacco was not harmful. Apologist scientists on the food-industry payroll continue to say that MSG is not harmful. They are better funded than those consumers, researchers, and physicians trying to spread the alarm. Public relations efforts include industry-bankrolled groups, which purport to represent consumers' food safety concerns but exist to claim that medical evidence condemning MSG is inconclusive.

About thirty years ago, the giant tobacco companies realized that fewer people were smoking and diversified to an industry that consumers could not avoid, buying control over food processing in the United States. Therefore, it should not be surprising to see similar tactics, which had worked for so many years with cigarettes.

All that being said, I am not going to go into detail about all of the alleged bad and dangerous side-effects of MSG. There are toxicologists and consumer advocates attempting to alert the public about those issues. I will let these other voices argue the toxic effects of this family of additives with the food industry. My reason for telling you, the dieter, to avoid MSG and similar flavor-enhancers is based upon the very same science that the food processors use to justify it. Simply put, MSG works magnificently as a flavor-enhancer and in doing so, it becomes a diet-buster.

When MSG is added to poor quality food or to an

artificially flavored substitute for real food, it makes it taste much better. Try eating just one flavored chip or snack containing MSG. Just like they advertise, it really can be difficult to stop at just one. I am surprised that I have not come across cardboard with MSG added. The food-flavoring experts could probably make it quite tasty.

In fact, scientists in the 1960s first showed what a powerful diet-buster MSG was. Feeding similar food to two groups of animals, with only one group having MSG added, the MSG-eating animals ate more and ended up weighing more than their non-MSG counterparts. Food scientists have known about this research for forty years. More recent research paints a picture that is even worse. A group of German scientists took this research experiment one step further. After the MSG-fed animals had eaten more and gained weight, the scientist stopped adding MSG to their food, but that group continued to eat more and gain weight for months. That experiment illustrated how the effects of MSG-induced weight-gain continued and showed that the gain was not limited to the food to which MSG was added

Forgetting all the other alleged effects of MSG, this one issue should be enough to influence anyone needing either to lose weight or to protect his or her family. ***This additive that can make you eat more is reason enough to avoid MSG.***

Saying *"avoid MSG"* is easy but actually doing it is hard work. The reason that I labeled this section "avoid flavor enhancers" was that the food industry has gone to great lengths to hide MSG in many products. Although these flavor-enhancers all act the same way, the food industry has figured out many ways to fool the public into thinking that they are avoiding MSG. Our loose food regulations look at the letter of the law through the eyes of the food-additive industry while

73

avoiding the intent of the law to protect the public.

Once consumers started attempting to avoid foods containing MSG in the 1960s, the food industry has been intent on finding *"clean"* alternatives. *"Clean,"* in this context, is industry terminology which I have heard from food-additive representatives. ***It does not mean free of MSG.*** Instead, it means finding creative chemical ways to avoid having to say MSG on the label!

You need some explanation of how MSG works in your nervous system to understand how they can get away with this. Going back to the inventor, the chemist Ikeda had determined the chemical composition of MSG but had no idea why it worked. At that time, scientists recognized the four taste receptors (sweet, sour, bitter and salty) on the tongue. To explain the amazing result from MSG, Ikeda proposed the existence of an additional taste receptor variously called "unami" or "tasty."

The existence of nervous-system signaling chemicals or neurotransmitters was not known in Ikeda's time. Today, we know much more about monosodium glutamate. It is composed of an atom of sodium (as found in table salt) attached to a molecule of glutamate, which is also known as glutamic acid. Glutamic acid is a common amino acid, one of the building blocks of protein throughout nature. You eat amino acids all the time, but, in nature, most are bound within the structure of the proteins we eat, whether that protein is from animal or vegetable sources.

Various normal cooking or processing methods may modify or break down miniscule amounts of protein, but, for the most part, amino acids are not separated and freed up until the protein we eat is broken down in the digestive process. MSG, on the other hand, hits our taste receptors as soon as the food containing it reaches our mouths. MSG can also pass directly into our bodies through the tissues of our mouth, skipping much of the process of digestion.

Glutamic acid is extremely important to our nervous system, because it serves as a neurotransmitter, a chemical that sends messages from one nerve cell to another. Glutamate is found as a neurotransmitter sending signals between the nerve cells judging taste in our brain. These cells in our taste pathways can be falsely stimulated. This false stimulation of this important nervous system pathway is similar to the way that many other drugs work. Such false triggering of important brain pathways is how many drugs work, even heroin and cocaine. Glutamic acid, when freed up from natural protein, can be used as such a drug. Attaching it to an atom of sodium allows it to easily reach the nervous system pathways which tell us how much flavor a food contains. **It chemically turns up the volume of any taste that is actually present, making it taste more flavorful and creating a desire to eat more.**

Some food-industry funded scientists and food-writers focused on Ikeda's old idea of a finding a *"tasty" or "unami"* receptor within the nervous system. The food industry hopes that this idea will deflect attention from the drug-like effect of MSG and other additives. Publicizing scientific debate about where in the nervous system MSG works attempts to avoid the discussion of the devastating impact that it has had. This is just like the earlier discovery of other neurotransmitter effects. In the 1970s, brain scientists discovered that the receptor sites for the natural endorphins in our brain were the same sites hijacked by opium and heroin. This important scientific knowledge did not make heroin addiction and its devastating consequences any more normal.

Whether MSG works at specific *"unami"* receptor sites

or simply turns up the volume by overwhelming all glutamic acid pathways does not change the harm that it causes by causing you to overeat. There are other scientists, not employed by the food industry, more worried about the toxic consequences of MSG. Those scientists point to evidence that MSG may over-stimulate the glutamate-dependent nerve cells in our taste pathways. This idea, called the excitotoxin hypothesis, claims that such overloaded cells may suffer long-term damage, which has lasting effects, as in the laboratory animals that just kept eating.

Yet, for the purpose of dieting, none of this matters. Your issue is that MSG is the prototype for many flavor-enhancing additives that influence how much you eat. As the food industry has added chemicals to more and more products, you become the victim. Again, I advise you to **avoid MSG because it is a diet-buster**.

It is not easy avoiding MSG because government labeling regulations favor the synthetic food processors. Simply put, they allow food manufacturers to camouflage MSG. Although some products tell you they contain MSG *(provided you read the fine print in their ingredients list),* others go to great lengths to fool you. This *"clean labeling"* game has been going on for three decades.

MSG can be manufactured from a variety of processes. They all involve some method of breaking down a protein, whether animal or vegetable. As an example, you can ferment a broth of crushed vegetable, fish, or beef protein and let microbes break apart the protein into its various amino acids. Another way is to use a solution that is heavily salted and let the osmotic pressure from the heavily salted water cause hydrolysis. This means a breaking apart, which frees the amino acids, letting them combine with salt solution.

> ### *Honest Labeling is Consumer Protection.*
>
> The first national Pure Food and Drug Act became law in 1906, when Teddy Roosevelt was President. One provision mandated honest labeling. At that time, millions of American women had become addicted to various "tonics" sold for "female complaints." These tonics temporarily relieved their symptoms but were impossible to stop taking. They often contained highly addictive combinations of opium, cocaine, and alcohol, but the user had no idea of their contents. This law preceded strict drug control, but it was highly effective in stopping the epidemic.
>
> Once women realized what was in these potions, they stopped becoming victims. As sales plummeted, manufacturers had to change their formulas or go out of business.

These are over-simplified explanations of some complex methods devised by the food processing and flavoring industries over many years.

They help explain why food labeling regulations give the food processing industry tremendous latitude. If the food processor adds powder from a large chemical drum labeled MSG, it must say MSG on the label of the finished product. However, if they add the chemical brew from a tanker car filled with one of the broth products I just described, they might be able to label their product as containing something other than MSG, such as:

- hydrolyzed vegetable protein
- HVP
- hydrolyzed soy protein
- hydrolyzed corn protein
- vegetable broth
- vegetable protein
- yeast extract
- fermented soy product

Those are just a few of the many aliases that MSG can take. More MSG aliases are listed in Chart 8-1 on page 86. Each of these products contains MSG or a similar chemical. Some names sound incomprehensible while others sound perfectly innocent. Vegetable broth sounds like some hearty dish that your grandmother might cook. Of course, you might wonder what grandma's vegetable broth was doing in your can of cheap tuna fish!

Another problem with MSG is the dietary "salt" issue. We have been told for several decades that everyone should cut back on their use of salt. Actually, this advice should not be for everyone. Many people with kidney, heart, and blood pressure issues must stay on sodium-restricted diets. Whether this is good advice for everyone else is questionable, and certain other people get too little sodium.

However, the vast majority of Americans do get a large amount of sodium in their diets. The press and sometimes the government always say "salt," since chemically table salt is sodium chloride. However, salt is not the issue. It is the sodium portion that is. Often, people on such low-sodium diets are given potassium chloride, a healthier chemical form of salt, often called a salt substitute. Why is this important? Stop and think for a moment. Doctors and biological scientists understand that **sodium** is the issue, not "salt." Sodium is added to the food supply in any food containing *mono**sodium** glutamate.* If you are someone who has been told to reduce your "salt," try reducing your MSG.

These are just a few of the ways MSG can be hidden. This will continue to be a problem until there are adequate laws warning consumers about hidden or disguised additives. Look for foods that are clearly labeled as **"MSG-free"** or **"No MSG,"** but even then, read the label. Food companies continue to test their limits with the lax enforcement of labeling standards. Never trust the phrase *"No Added MSG,"* it is as misleading as *"No Added Sugar."*

Do not be surprised at the many places you find MSG hiding. It is common in snack foods such as chips and coated nuts. It shows up in canned ravioli, seasoned french fries, frozen dinners, and in canned tuna fish. It is common in many restaurants and is sometimes found in the *"seasoned salts"* served at restaurants and perhaps found on your spice rack. After you begin to read labels closely, you should suspect it everywhere!

Avoiding Engineered Fats

Dietary fat has been given a bad reputation that it does not deserve. The type of fat you eat is more important than how much fat you eat. All people need fat in their diet, because although your body can create storage fat from extra energy, you need a few types of fats, called "essential fatty acids." These can only come from what you eat. On this diet, keeping the right proportion and amount of fat in your diet is an absolute necessity, because it is the trigger to burn up your stored fat. At the same time, it makes sense to distinguish good from bad fats, while you are changing your habits and lifestyle of many years.

Food scientists have used selective breeding, genetic engineering, chemical modification, and other methods to create substitutes for the healthiest fats. Try to avoid all of these engineered substitutes. Natural fats such as olive oil have been keeping people healthy since biblical times.

Later, we will discuss picking the very best fats, including those high in omega-3 fatty acids, such as those found in certain fish and those very high in monounsaturated fat, such as olive oil. Many people believe that all saturated fat is bad, but that is not the case. A diet with a reasonable amount of natural saturated fat found in dairy, meat, and poultry is perfectly healthy.

What are the unhealthiest fats? They are the artificially modified vegetable fats called *hydrogenated* or *trans*-fats. About a century ago, chemists discovered that if they took some of the very cheapest vegetable oils and chemically modified them through a process known as *hydrogenation,* they could thicken them and change their appearance and cooking characteristics. One of the first uses for these hydrogenated fats was in the baking industry. Hydrogenated fats were cheap and easy to use as substitutes for the butter or lard typically used as shortening in fine pastry.

Another use was for margarine, but initially, the public was not easily fooled by this cheap substitute. The typical margarine is made from an inexpensive vegetable oil, which has been synthetically hardened by hydrogenation. Hydrogenated fat produces a grayish-white substance that had no resemblance to butter. Dye is added to produce a butter-like color. Food shortages in both World War I and II created a temporary market for this inferior product, but people understood that it was a cheap substitute for the real product, butter.

Some states, particularly those with dairy industries, put legal restrictions on the sale and use of margarine. These restrictions were aimed at protecting the public from being sold these products without their knowledge. Today, these restrictions are all gone. Misinterpretation of scientific data beginning in the 1950s and 1960s led the public to believe that margarine was healthier than butter, since it was made from vegetable oil. The industry conveniently forgot to tell the public that, once vegetable oil had been hydrogenated, it not only resembled saturated fat but did so in an unnatural and unhealthy way.

Canned vegetable shortening was sold to homemakers and began to replace butter and lard for frying and home baking. Companies also *"partially hydrogenated"* liquid vegetable oils because hydrogenation also slows the rate at which oils turn rancid. This was important to the fast-food industry, since they typically keep large amounts of oil in open fryers for many days.

The public is just beginning to understand what chemists and physicians have known for a century. This hydrogenation process bonds together molecules in an unnatural way. These bonds face in the opposite direction of natural fats. They are called *trans*-fats, from the Latin word for "across." This is because the bonds holding these fat chains together cut across in this opposite direction. Unfortunately, our bodies do not deal well with this excess of backward-facing fat. As these fats are broken down, these oddly-bonded fragments end up creating health problems.

These hydrogenated or *trans*-fats are the real villains. People have been eating healthy natural fat for millennia. It is only in the last century that our food supply has been modified with this cheap substitute. **Never eat any food with the word *hydrogenated* in the ingredients list!**

Another unusual type of ingredient is sometimes called tropical oil, or may it be listed as vegetable oil, palm-kernel oil or coconut oil. These oils, grown on a plantation in tropical climates, have an unusual characteristic, for although they are vegetable in origin, they contain a high degree of saturated fat, like meat and butterfat. Typically, they are then hydrogenated and used in cheap commercial baked goods. Again, always stay away from hydrogenated oil. In general, there is little good to be said for palm-kernel oil, but coconut oil has a special characteristic that some people may need. We discussed this with the information about MCT oils in Chapter 5.

What about fats that have been modified in other ways? That is a tough call. Today, plant scientists and genetic engineers are trying to manipulate vegetable oils that have been around forever. They are doing so to try to get these cheap vegetable oils to resemble some of the healthiest oils. This is a noble goal, but is it a good choice for you? The jury is still out on these manipulations of the food chain. If you can afford the admittedly high price of real olive oil, do you want to save a few pennies by buying a cheaper vegetable oil that has been manipulated to be " almost as good as olive oil"?

Going Sugar-Free

Going sugar-free is one of the healthiest things you can do, no matter what type of diet you follow. Sugar should be eaten only in context, that is, in the way sugar is found in nature. For thousands of years, purified sugar was a relative rarity. It was considered a luxury. The main source of pure sugar was wild honey. Foods that were naturally high in sugar were not year-around foods. Typically, high-sugar foods such as fruit could be eaten only during a brief season. Otherwise, they would have to be preserved by drying, such as turning grapes into raisins, or they would naturally ferment to alcohol or vinegar.

Sugar extraction was developed in India more than two thousand years ago, but the process was a guarded secret, which spread very slowly to the rest of the world. Sugar was considered a rare spice and consumed in small quantities by the rich or royalty. Even then, doctors noted diseases associated with the beginning of sugar consumption.

The greatest change in human sugar consumption came about with the European colonization of tropical regions. The European nations used slave labor to mass produce sugar cane, turning a rarity into a cheap product. Human consumption of sugar has been growing steadily since that time. Beet sugar and corn syrup have been developed as even cheaper substitute sources of sugar.

Today, the developing countries are getting hooked on high-sugar soft drinks and sweets. Indeed, the growth of sugar consumption in the newly industrialized world has led to an epidemic of obesity in countries such as India and China, nations where we still picture starvation and malnutrition. Ironically, they are now plagued by both obesity and malnutrition, not in the same people, but side-by-side, as they move from poor agricultural economies to Western-style manufacturing economies!

In both people and animals, such sugar use is unnatural. This heavy year-around use of sugar is addictive, because in addition to tasting good, this over-use of sugar has set up bodily changes so that you constantly want to maintain a high-carbohydrate consumption level.. One of the most difficult issues in reducing sugar consumption is the acquired taste that the human race has developed in the past several hundred years. As you diet, your taste for sweets will diminish. As long as you keep away from the sugar rush, your taste for sweets will gradually change. In the meantime, use sugar substitutes. This will separate the taste craving that you have long associated with the sugar rush.

This means avoiding all food to which sugar has been added. This seems tough, until you have been weaned from the linkage between the sugar taste and the sugar rush. Fortunately, there are many acceptable sugar substitutes. A debate has gone on for decades regarding potential health risks of sugar substitutes. More will be said on sugar substitutes in the next chapter. Remember, the debate about supposed harm from sugar substitutes is largely hypothetical, but the health risk from sugar is real and devastating. Do not be afraid of sugar substitutes, be very afraid of sugar.

Many foods contain hidden sugar. Avoid all foods that claim that they contain half the sugar or light sugar. They are simply stating that they use less sugar than a worse product, often by combining artificial sweetener with real sugar. Always read the nutritional label to be sure that zero calories are listed under sugar.

The Food and Drug Administration requires that ingredients listed on the label should be in order of quantity. That means that if the greatest proportion of ingredients is sugar that should come first on the label. Manufacturers have figured a clever way to trick the public. By using two or three different types of sugar, although the total would be first on a label, the individual sugars are not listed first; they are hidden down in the list of ingredients. Another trick is to use chemical names for common sugars, hoping that you, the consumer will not recognize this. Such names include sucrose, dextrose, lactose, glucose, fructose and many other chemical names ending in "ose." *Treat every "ose" name as just another sugar.*

Another food industry trick is to use concentrates that make pure sugar sound like a healthy natural food. Examples are corn syrup and fruit juice concentrate. We think of fruit juice as natural and healthy, so the food companies use this ploy to stuff children's drinks with inexpensive apple-juice concentrate from China. They then have the nerve to say *"no added sugar"* boldly on the label!

Corn syrup is a another cheap source of very pure sugar and modified corn syrup is a substance that has been changed to make it taste even sweeter. More than one food company lists *"refined cane extract"* as an ingredient on their label. Translated into plain English, *"refined cane extract"* is actually ordinary table sugar!

As you have been reading this chapter, you may have been feeling that points I have been making were exaggerated. I would not blame you, for many of my patients have wondered this until their next trip to the grocery. Once they begin to read labels closely, they are amazed at what went into supposedly healthy food that they thought they had been purchasing. Now, they are all devoted and somewhat paranoid label-readers.

Read all food labels suspiciously!

Chart 8-1

Many Names of Hidden Glutamate Flavor Enhancers

Certainly or Probably Contains MSG

Autolyzed "anything"
Autolyzed plant protein
Autolyzed yeast
Calcium caseinate
Disodium inosinate
Disodium guanylate
DSG
DSI
Glutamate
Glutamic acid
HPP
HVP

Hydrolyzed "anything"
Hydrolyzed corn protein
Hydrolyzed soy protein
Hydrolyzed plant protein
Hydrolyzed vegetable protein
Monopotassium glutamate
Monosodium glutamate
Sodium caseinate
Textured protein
Vegetable broth
Yeast extract
Yeast food or nutrient

Possibly Contains or Associated with MSG

Annatto
Barley malt
Broth, stock or bouillon
Caramel flavoring or coloring
Carrageenan
Citric acid (when processed from corn)
Corn syrup and corn syrup solids
Cornstarch
Dough conditioners
Fermented "anything"
Flavors, flavoring, seasonings, "spices", extract, reaction flavors
Flowing agents
Gelatin (except gelatin desserts)
Gums
Lipolyzed butter fat
"Low" or "No-fat" items
Malted barley
Maltodextrin

Modified "anything"
Modified food starch
Natural chicken, beef, or pork flavoring
Pectin enzymes
Protease
Protease enzymes
Protein-fortified milk, whey-protein, whey, milk powder, dry milk solids, whey protein isolate or concentrate
Protein-fortified "anything"
Rice syrup
Soy, wheat, rice, or oat protein
Soy sauce or extract
Soy-protein isolate or concentrate
Ultra-pasteurized "anything"

Or
Any Ingredients that Appear Out of Place
for the Food They Are In

Going Shopping

The key to this diet being effective is being very aware of what you eat. The simpler and healthier the ingredients you use, the better off you are. Allow more time for your shopping. As you begin to scrutinize the food you purchase, you will find that reading labels takes time. Gradually, as you discover what items to trust and what to avoid, your shopping trips will return to normal. Until then, keep reminding yourself to read both the ingredients list and the nutritional labeling to discover what you are really eating. Here are a number of simple rules to help you:

- *Avoid all sugars*
- *Fresher is always better*
- *Ignore phony health claims*
- *Do not trust the word "natural" without proof*
- *Avoid ingredients you do not understand*
- *Pick the product with the shortest ingredient list*
- *Do not be afraid to spend a little more for better foods*
- *Learn what foods you enjoy on this diet and use them*

There are some federal regulations about how food processing companies have to structure their labels. Although they try to be "creative," they have to adhere to a certain style in these labels. It is important that you learn how to read this important information. You may know some of these conventions but others may be a revelation to you.

There is always an ingredients list. The exception is for some products with only a single ingredient. As an example, a spice labeled *"black pepper"* might not have an ingredients list but a spice labeled *"seasoned pepper,"* which contains multiple ingredients would need an ingredients list. All ingredients are listed in order of quantity. Therefore, the first ingredient on the list is present in the largest quantity while the last ingredient is there in the smallest quantity.

Many consumers already know this. Some shoppers who want to avoid high sugar foods try not to buy foods where sugar is listed as the first ingredient. Food companies know this and deliberately avoid placing sugar first on the label, particularly for children's items. As we discussed previously, the way that they do this is devious but perfectly legal. Instead of using one type of sugar, they may mix two, three, even four separate types of sugar. This brings the percentage of each type down so that another ingredient takes first place on the label.

Look for short ingredient lists. Generally, the purer the food, the fewer the number of ingredients, so longer lists often spell trouble. Look for any of the hidden or suspicious forms for MSG. Be suspicious of ingredients you do not recognize. One dieter recently told me "since starting this diet, I do not buy any food with ingredients that I cannot pronounce." That is some pretty sound advice. Although it may make you avoid some foods with innocent ingredients, it will prevent many mistakes.

Do not forget that the government allows many different names for the same ingredient. This freedom allows ridiculous attempts to fool the consumer. An example is one product where the first ingredient listed is *"evaporated cane juice."* Juice sounds healthy, does it not? If you pause a moment to think, you will realize the *"cane"* is sugar cane. **That means evaporated cane juice is just plain old sugar.**

Do not be content just because you recognize the names of everything. Pause a moment and question why an ingredient is there. Words like gelatin or broth can be innocent enough in the right context or they can be deceptive ways of describing ingredients you wish to avoid. Be suspicious when you notice something that does not seem to belong. Be suspicious of the word natural, as in **"natural flavoring"** or **"natural coloring."** Do not forget that the FDA considers creepy-crawlies to be natural, as in allowing crushed red beetle juice to be called *"natural coloring"* for strawberry yogurt!

Some people advise "shopping around the perimeter of the supermarkets" to find the purer foods. There is truth to this advice, but it is often not sufficient. What they mean by shopping around the perimeter is to totally avoid all the processed foods. The perimeter or wall of a typical supermarket often contains the produce department, the dairy case, and the meat and fish departments. Unfortunately, the dairy case also contains artificial creamers, dairy products altered with faux ingredients, and similar items. The meat department may contain meat and poultry injected with flavor-enhancing broth. The fish department may contain frozen pre-seasoned fish loaded with MSG.

Despite all this negative advice, you will quickly become quite positive about shopping. Once you know how to determine what is good and bad for your diet, you will no longer have to read dozens of labels in the store. Just be prepared for a long visit the first time or two that you go to the supermarket.

This is an example of an actual "Nutrition Facts" box followed by an explanation of how to use it. After the ingredients list, it is the second most important piece of information on any packaged food. Read the explanation to learn about the key areas pointed to by the numbered arrows.

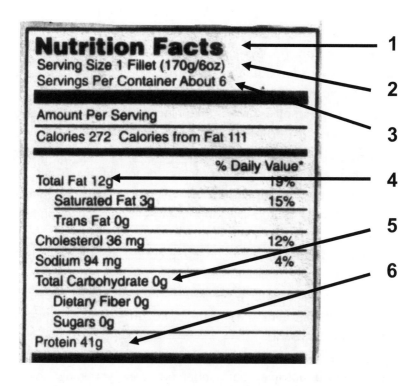

The New Hippocratic Diet

1. The box is headed by the words "Nutrition Facts" in large bold print. Most products contain this box. The only exception is for a product in a very small package such as candy or gum. If there is not enough room to use the box format, the manufacturer will sometimes provide the same information in a textual format, usually in extremely fine print.

2. The next line explains the serving size. In this case, it is an individual fish fillet weighing approximately six ounces.

3. The next line tells you how many servings are in this package. In this case, there are six frozen fish fillets in one container. Be careful here. There are some items that are sold as individual portions; yet, the label says that the container has multiple portions. One notorious example is individual vending machine bottles of cola that are clearly sold for individual use; yet, the label shows multiple servings. This enables the manufacturer to imply lower calorie counts per serving than is actually the case.

4. Total fat is the first major category. In this case, the serving of fish contains twelve grams of total fat. The subheadings showing the type of fat are sometimes useful in understanding more about the food item, but they are often incomplete. Ignore the column labeled percentage daily value.

5. The next item of importance to you is total carbohydrate. In this case, the fish contains no carbohydrates, which is generally good for this diet. There may be additional subheadings under this category, which we will explain shortly.

6. Protein is the next significant item. In this case, the fish contains forty-one grams of protein in this single filet.

If you were considering this for dinner, note one slight problem. You remember the 60-40-10 suggestions? This single fish fillet contains your entire day's worth of protein. Unless you were only having one meal that day, this would not be a wise choice. The solution is simple. Go back to the serving size and halve it, so that you only have three ounces of fish. Then it becomes an entirely appropriate portion.

When reading these charts, be watchful, for there may be hidden items. For example, a product's ingredients list may show that it contains sugar yet the "Nutrition Facts" may state that it contains zero grams of sugar and zero calories from sugar. What is happening? The government regulations allow the manufacturer to round down, so a product with less than one gram of sugar might say zero, while it actually contains a small amount. This may or may not be important to you, depending on how much you actually plan to use. If the ingredients list says it contains sugar, take it into account and add a small amount in your calculations.

Keep in mind that anything outside the ingredients list and Nutrition Facts box is subject to a different set of rules. Lawyers and advertisers use the term "*puffery.*" Legally, puffery refers to fanciful statements that are made to make a product sound good. They are often exaggerated facts or "puffed up" features about a product. The only time the government regulators step in is when they decide these statements are harmful.

Often, a competitor will make a complaint to the government, feeling that exaggerated claims give its competitor an unfair advantage in the marketplace. One example might be a food product that claimed it could prevent cancer. A competitor could complain and government regulators could rule that making such a health claim was wrong. On the other hand, if the government became convinced that the food manufacturers had done nothing wrong and allowed them to continue, their competitor would feel that they had to make similar claims to maintain their share of the market. Although such claims may seem outlandish, they may be half-truths. Claims like this are not as tough to make as claims made on a new medicine.

A pharmaceutical manufacturer claiming that a drug might treat or prevent cancer would have to spend hundreds of millions of dollars testing and proving this to the satisfaction of government regulators. On the other hand, an advertising department that learned that one ingredient in a particular food might help in some health problem has a far lower standard to meet. Many products appear on the market with puffery on the front of the label that imply they will make you healthier, thinner, prettier, and smarter. Treat those claims for what they are.

An oddity about food labels is that they must contain information about nutrients that your body will not use. As an example, fiber that is not digestible by people is still chemically a carbohydrate. The government regulations require that these carbohydrates be included in the total carbohydrates shown. However, they can then be shown under the subheading of "Fiber" and you are supposed to know enough to subtract this. Perhaps the expert genius who thought this up was mixing up people with cows, since cows are able to digest this fiber.

Another subtraction should be done for "*sugar alcohols*," the chemical name for a group of substances that are neither what you would commonly think of as either sugar or alcohol. Instead, these are chemicals that should be treated as artificial sweeteners, but with a peculiar twist. They resemble sugar in the molecular region that matches our taste buds, so that you taste them as sugar but they do not match closely enough for your digestive system to use. If you see the term "sugar alcohol" in the Nutrition Facts box, once again, you subtract. You may also recognize them in the ingredients list, if you see a name ending in the letters *"ol,"* such as *"sorbitol."*

Here is an example of what you must do when seeing either sugar alcohol or fiber listed in the carbohydrate section. This example is from a label for a sugar-free candy.

Nutrition Facts

Serving Size 3 pieces (43g)
Serving Per Container about 2

Total Fat   12 g

Total Carbohydrate 24 g
   Dietary Fiber 2g
   Sugars 0g
   Sugar Alcohol 22 g

Protein 2g

In this case, you may subtract both the fiber (2 grams) and sugar alcohol (22 grams) from the total, resulting in 0 grams net carbohydrate! The same regulations that prevent the manufacturer from showing this accurately in the "Nutrition Facts" box do allow the company to brag about it on the front of the package. Depending upon whether they are marketing to dieters or to others, they <u>may</u> chose to advertise this as "Net Carbs" on the front of the package. You will find these sorts of statements on <u>some</u> lines of diet candy and ice cream, but there is little consistency.

Before you get too excited at the thought of candy and ice cream that you may eat on this diet, there is a down-side. Bacteria digest sugar alcohol. All those sugar-alcohol carbohydrates that your body cannot digest end up in your large intestine, where your normal intestinal bacteria feast on them. As a result, if you have more than a little, you may get gas and diarrhea as you overdo these sugar-free treats. People seem to differ in how much they can tolerate, so please be careful. Just because the package says a serving is three pieces, you do not have to follow that. If you try a product like this, start with just one.

Now, begin your trip through your local supermarket. Walk in the door and turn right toward produce. The fresh fruits will have to wait until you level off at your maintenance phase. Instead, head for the vegetables. Stock up on head lettuce in any variety you like. You may want fresh spinach for salad or cooking. Prepackaged lettuce mixtures are fine, provided they do not include any flavorings or dressings. You may want some celery for dips. Red and green peppers are a good choice to add some flavor to your cooking. Broccoli and asparagus are more good choices in the vegetable section. Cauliflower will be very useful to you, even if you do not eat it now, because it is found in some recipes as a potato substitute. You may be skeptical about that but once you have tried the recipes, you will understand why people often prefer it. If you like coleslaw, shredded cabbage is okay in moderation, but do not use it for a large vegetable course. Skip the starchy foods, such as beans, potatoes and beets.

If there is an olive bar in the vegetable department and you like olives, they are a welcome addition to this diet. Canned olives are good, too. The Manzanilla variety of olives are high in healthy olive oil.

Tomatoes are high in carbohydrates, so use them sparingly. Purchasing grape tomatoes is one way to control the amount you eat, since you can just use one or two as a flavoring on your salad. Onions contain carbohydrates, so if you use them in cooking, limit yourself to small amounts for flavoring. Try to avoid caramelizing them in cooking, as that turns their starch into sugar. Carrots are carbohydrate-containing root vegetables, so do not buy regular-size carrots. If you want to use them as a dip or a garnish, get those small, pre-peeled baby carrots and use and them in moderation.

Next, move to the section where salad dressings and toppings are sold. If you use a bacon-like topping on your salad, switch to the real thing and be sure it is MSG-free. Salad dressings are going to be much tougher. You will be very disappointed as you read the ingredients list, because most of the bottled salad dressings contain MSG, sugar, or both. The powdered salad dressing spice mixtures that you mix with your own oil and vinegar are usually no better than the bottled products.

A salad dressing should be essentially free of carbohydrate, so read the Nutrition Facts box. If your market has a section containing refrigerated salad dressings, you may have better luck. You will probably end up using some of the homemade salad dressings from the recipes we have given you or using simple oil and vinegar on your salads.

This is a good time to stop and buy vinegar. Ordinary white vinegar is nutrient free, while other vinegars, such as wine, malt or cider vinegar may contain traces of carbohydrate. Avoid balsamic vinegar, since it is made by mixing wine vinegar with *grape must*, a form of concentrated grape juice which adds a significant amount of carbohydrate.

Next, move on to the oil section. As you have probably already guessed, I am going to suggest that you stock up on the "extra-virgin" grade of olive oil. It is the best all-around type of oil that you can use. If you do a significant amount of deep-frying, you probably already have some peanut oil. It is fine for this purpose. If your market carries it, pick up some unrefined sesame oil to try on your salads. You may have to look in the gourmet foods department or go to a health food store to find this product. Try to avoid soybean oil, cotton seed oil and anything generically labeled "vegetable oil." Avoid all products labeled "shortening."

Find the spice aisle. Here you can experiment with a variety of spices that you may not have tried before. Virtually all pure spices are fine on this diet. Spice mixtures require more caution so read all of the ingredients list. Many mixtures contain MSG and some contain sugar. There are some excellent mixtures that will add a spirit to your cooking without any MSG or sugar. You will be amazed at the way real spices can bring out the flavor of real food without artificial flavor enhancers. Some recipes in this book call for items popular in Latin America, such as chipotle sauce and other spices. Many markets today have a separate ethnic food section where you can find these.

If you are near the condiment section, look for a real mayonnaise in a brand that you like. *Real mayonnaise* is one of those regulated names and must contain proper amounts of oil and eggs. Beyond that, it may contain a lot of other unnecessary ingredients. Check the ingredients and go for the shorter list. Unfortunately, most mayonnaise on the market today is made from soybean oil, not the best choice but a necessary compromise in many cases. If you can afford it, you might find a far more expensive mayonnaise made from all olive all oil in the gourmet section. Once again, read the label carefully, so that you do not waste extra money on a product where they add a few drops of olive oil to ordinary mayonnaise.

There is another mayonnaise choice. Gourmet cookbooks contain recipes for homemade mayonnaise using olive oil. However, I advise against this unless you can find salmonella-free eggs. Egg farms today are mass-production centers that are breeding grounds for salmonella bacteria in the laying hens. The eggs they produce are safe to eat only if completely cooked. Factory-made mayonnaise is safe because it is sterilized in the bottling process but homemade mayonnaise is not. There is a new process that will destroy salmonella in raw eggs, allowing their safe use. Those treated eggs can now be found only at one supermarket chain and one wholesale restaurant supplier, but check our website www.HippocraticDiet.com for newer information. Until then, compromise on the mass-produced store-bought mayonnaise.

Since you still are in the condiments section, you may want to pick up some pickles or some pickle relish. If you do, read the labels closely and avoid the ones sweetened with sugar.

If you are interested in mustard, most prepared mustards are okay except for the sweetened varieties with added sugar. If you crave the taste of sweetened mustard, add some calorie-free sweetener to prepared mustard.

Are you a ketchup user? Tomatoes do have natural carbohydrates, but most brands of ketchup also contain large amounts of added sugar or high fructose corn syrup. Low-carb ketchup is now available, if you wish.

Avoid the barbecue and steak sauces. Instead, use the calorie-free barbecue sauce recipe found in the recipe section of Chapter 14. It is made from smoked chipotle pepper sauce and works well for both steaks and barbecue.

Skip the Worcestershire sauce family entirely. The classic form of Worcestershire sauce contains fermented anchovies. This is one of the few historic forms of free glutamate, or MSG. The newer, cheaper Worcestershire sauces usually contain the chemical form of MSG. Either way, you lose.

You may find the baking and sweetening section nearby. Look for the artificial sweeteners we mentioned earlier. If you do not like artificial sweeteners, consider Stevia, a calorie-free sweetener from an herb. Pick up some unsweetened 100 percent pure baking cocoa. Do not forget to stock up on liquid non-calorie sweetener. You may also wish to buy a non-calorie brown sugar substitute, but you must be careful when purchasing non-calorie sweeteners. There is at least one well-known brand that uses its brand name on both non-calorie and reduced-calorie sweeteners, so you must read every label and not just rely on a familiar brand name.

You may prefer to get your vegetables in the frozen food or canned food departments. Both are fine, if you are buying pure vegetables. However, be cautious and avoid vegetables with added ingredients. Look out for sugar that is added to certain canned vegetables. In the frozen vegetable department, stay away from vegetables that come with added sauces and, of course, mixtures containing beans, peas or pasta.

Next, you may be ready to visit the meat department of your market. If you live in a big city, you might be lucky enough to find some local independent butcher shops nearby. If you live near a rural area, a local farmer, rancher or packing plant may sell locally raised meat products without injected additives.

Otherwise, you are stuck with the large big-box supermarket with its so-called meat department. I say "so-called" because there is a trend for supermarkets to use prepackaged meats. Peek behind the freezer case wall. See if there are people in white coats cutting large sections of meat into small slices or if they are simply opening large cartons of pre-processed food. Try to avoid the chain markets that have their meat cut and packaged in the large processing plants.

Whatever you do, do not buy your meat in those pre-cut restaurant and individual serving packages, whether it is from a supermarket, a home delivery service, or by a mail order. Such portion-controlled meat is highly likely to be infused with a broth that is a devil's brew of free glutamates, preservatives, and other chemicals. They even go so far as to douse their meats with deadly carbon monoxide gas, which prevents the blood in the meat from turning brown and allows old meat to retain a fresh red appearance.

Do not be fooled by advertising that a particular meat product is hormone-free or antibiotic-free. Those are nice attributes providing information about how the animals were raised, but they tell you nothing about what chemicals were added by the meat processor. I have seen packing plants selling "Amish-raised meats" where MSG-containing spice mixtures were added to ground sausage. Even products passing the rigorous religious inspection process for a kosher meat certification may have MSG-containing hydrolyzed vegetable protein added.

Poultry can be just as bad as other products. Fresh poultry markets were once common but are a rarity today. Most poultry sold in supermarkets has been processed hundreds or thousands of miles from where it is being sold. It is then infused with another magic broth. There is one national brand which costs a lot more that is free of this broth. It is worth the extra price and it is a tastier product than the modified chicken, but be careful. The food-processing companies know a good thing when they see it. They now sell alternative, supposedly premium brands of poultry right next to this expensive brand. Their supposedly premium chicken may have all sorts of puffery and claims on the front label but turn it over and you will see that it contains the same magic broth as the cheaper chicken. When you are paying a premium price, you deserve the real product for which you pay extra.

Seafood is another matter. Its hard say which seafood alternative is better. Today, some fish is frozen and sealed at large South American ocean-side fish farms, inland Asian fish farms, or massive foreign refrigerator ships. Other fish is cut and sold at your local supermarket fish counter but usually is no fresher. Most often, those products are simply frozen whole, then thawed at your supermarket before they are put on ice and sold as if fresh. The old-fashioned fish market where fresh products were sold is a rarity, except for a few costal areas where fishing fleets operate.

Remember that the darker the fish, the higher the percentage of healthy fish oil. Shellfish such as crab and lobster is okay, but contains little or no fat. That is why it is so traditional to dip lobster meat in drawn butter. Stay away from the imitation crab and lobster meat. This is usually a cheap whitefish such as pollack or cod, which has been infused with artificial flavoring and MSG.

Canned fish may be okay, depending on what it is. You can get sardines packed in oil without additives. You may want canned kippered herring, which is high in healthy fish oil. Canned salmon works well in some recipes. Avoid fermented anchovies because of the possibility of free glutamate.

Canned tuna is a special case. Healthy tuna packed in olive oil is still available in supermarkets but it is hard to find. Years ago, at the beginning of the low-fat craze, the food companies convinced many people to switch to lighter tuna packed in water. Consumers did so in the mistaken belief that it was a healthier choice. The packers were actually substituting a cheaper variety of fish for the better quality darker tuna. To give it flavor they pack it in hydrolyzed vegetable broth. The real stuff, when you can find it, is sold as a gourmet premium product at about three times the cost of the cheapest canned tuna, but It is worth paying extra for. Read the ingredients list carefully. It should list only tuna and olive oil. If you normally use canned tuna only as an ingredient in tuna salad, you will be pleasantly surprised. MSG-free tuna in olive oil is delicious right out of the can. Adding a bit of this canned tuna to a green salad makes a tasty and well-balanced meal.

Since meat products may still be on your mind, let us talk about the delicatessen section. The deli section can be found in two places. There are the inexpensive prepackaged processed sliced meat products in a refrigerator case, then there is the deli counter where they will slice better quality products to your order.

Surprisingly, I must tell you to avoid the deli counter, unless you have a good relationship with the workers there. The prepackaged products in the refrigerator case all have labels that you can read. The bulk products at the deli counter have labels on the bulk packages, but asking to see each of the labels at a busy deli counter can be a real problem. I have tried, without success, to get this information directly from the food producers. Even though it is not a secret and is readily available to the people behind the counter, these companies would still rather not have you read their labels. This is sad, since many of these producers portray an image of purity and wholesomeness. You would think they would not try to keep this information from your eyes.

If you do buy deli products from the refrigerator case, at least you can take your time and read the fine print of the ingredient label. Very few of these products are free of MSG or hydrolyzed vegetable protein or some other form of free-glutamate. The few that are MSG-free often boast of it on the front label, but you still want to double-check the ingredient list. Some producers are not above saying *MSG-free* on the front of the package while the ingredient list clearly shows hydrolyzed vegetable protein. Others resort to extreme trickery, such as the company that boasts "*No added MSG * * *" on its front label. The words *NO* and *MSG* are highlighted while the word *added* is in small print. You have to search the entire package until you find the * * explained in a footnote at the bottom of the package back in very fine print. It reads " * * *except that found naturally in hydrolyzed vegetable protein.*" Of course, the ingredient list does list the hydrolyzed vegetable protein. *What is the average consumer to think?*

If you look hard enough, you will find a few products that are truly MSG-free, but it takes some work. Many of the cured products, such as ham and bacon, also contain sugar. Try to find the ones with the least amount of sugar, using the Nutrition Facts box.

Cured meat products may also contain preservatives, such as nitrate. These preservatives serve an important function by protecting food from dangerous bacterial spoilage. Unfortunately, some believe they can cause other health problems. This is another one of those areas where you must weigh one health issue against another. It is too lengthy a topic to cover here and does not relate to the obesity issue.

However, for those of you who wish to avoid nitrates, be warned. Many food products boast that they do not contain nitrates but, in fact, they use substitute additives that turn into nitrate after being added to food. *It seems as if truth-in-labeling has a long way to go!*

Leaving the deli department. do not forget to shop for dairy products. Traditionally, it had always been the butterfat-containing cream that was recognized as the most significant milk product. An old name for a milk-processing facility was *creamery*. It was the important cream portion that was vital for the nutritionally rich butter and cheese products. When completely separated, the left-over skim milk portion had other historic uses. These have included being the base for house paint and used as hog feed or slop.

Sorry, but while dieting, you should avoid whole milk. Instead, the first thing on your list should be heavy whipping cream. If your market carries it, the best type of whipping cream is pure and fresh. Unfortunately, this can be difficult to find.

Recently, creameries switched to producing ultra-pasteurized cream. The reason for this was pure economics. Ultra-pasteurization is a process that heats the product to a slightly higher temperature than regular pasteurization. This allows the finished product to have a longer shelf life while refrigerated and some products do not need any refrigeration. These ultra-pasteurized products last for months before spoiling. The disadvantage of this method is that the flavor of the product is altered. To compensate, the producers may add various flavor enhancers. Some producers go one step further, also adding thickeners and coloring agents and including less cream in the product. When buying cream, follow the shorter-list rule. If you can find it, buy fresh cream that has been pasteurized but not ultra-pasteurized. If you cannot find this pure product, buy the cream with the shortest ingredient list.

If you wish, buy butter. Avoid butter substitutes. Salted butter is the purest product. Unsalted sweet butter may contain extra additives.

Cheese should be the next item on your list. Whether it comes in a block, sliced, cubed, shredded or grated, real cheese is made with cream, enzymes, and perhaps salt. Sometimes annatto is added for a bright orange color. Some of the grated and shredded cheeses have small amounts of other ingredients added as flowing agents. These flowing agents sometimes contain small amounts of carbohydrate.

Some recipes call for crumpled bleu cheese or feta cheese. If you prefer, you can purchase this product whole and crumble it yourself. By doing this, you will avoid the carbohydrate-containing flowing agent added to the pre-crumbled cheese. The same goes for shredded cheese that ordinarily comes in a shaker box.

Avoid items called *imitation cheese* or *cheese-products*. They are usually made by substituting vegetable oils for the real cream and may be loaded with other products. Read the Nutrition Facts box and ingredient list on any cheese that you buy.

Cheese is a healthy and nutritious food that has been in use for millennia. It took a beating from the low-fat craze but it is making a comeback. It will be useful in a number of recipes. Cheese cubes are also a handy snack food. One small caution about eating cheese. Some people will find that they become constipated when they eat too much cheese. If this happens to you, modify your cheese intake.

Real sour cream is another important product. When you compare the ingredient list on real sour cream to the various imitation forms of light or non-fat sour cream, you will see the difference. The Nutrition Facts boxes will show quite a remarkable contrast, too. There are a number of important recipes that you will find in this book calling for real sour cream. Stock up on it early, since it is allowed during the initiation phase.

Eggs are usually found nearby. Stock up on them. It is amazing that eggs went from being a health food, with the U.S. government recommending that you eat one egg every day to a taboo food with the government recommending that you avoid eggs. They are now back to being a health food and you will even find premium eggs with the chickens fed in a way that increases their eggs' content of healthy omega-3 fatty acid.

As you leave the dairy department, you may want to visit the beverage department and snack department on your way to the check-out cashier. In the beverage department, coffee, tea, and herbal tea are fine. Avoid the pre-mixed flavored instant coffees and teas that often contain sugar. Avoid any powdered beverage unless it clearly is labeled as zero calories.

If you are a soda drinker, this diet allows reasonable amounts of non-calorie diet soda. Although there are other health concerns with these products, I am not restricting their use for the purposes of this diet. There is even one recipe for "real cream soda" in this book, mixing a small amount of real cream and diet soda. It is a useful thing to try during the initiation phase and many non-soda drinkers love it, since it tastes like an old-fashioned ice cream float.

Non-calorie flavored seltzer and sparkling water are allowed. It is even okay to use those Italian-style flavoring syrups they use in the coffee shops if you can find the sugar-free variety. Despite saying it is permitted to use this wide range of non-calorie beverages, the best beverage is always water. Drink water liberally. If the tap water in your area has an off-taste, consider purchasing bottled water or using a water-filtering pitcher.

Snacks might seem incompatible with dieting, but they are important. Finding satisfying snacks that stay within the limits of this diet gives you the ability to handle special situations. Treat snacks like any other food item. Keep track of them because quantity counts!

One of the best group of foods that are found in the snack section are nuts. These include the true tree nuts, seeds such as sunflower and pumpkin, and peanuts which are actually related to peas and beans. All of them contain a mixture of fat, protein, and carbohydrates. In modest quantities, they are all acceptable on this diet but if you overdo it, you may exceed your carbohydrate allowance.

Many dieters love roasted cashews and almonds but many have issues with portion control when eating these delicious but healthy snacks. One of the best ways around this is to buy nuts in small bags instead of large cans. Another way that works well is to use small plastic snack bags and measure out the proper amount in advance.

Portion control is easier if you can buy nuts still in the shell. Pistachios, peanuts, and sunflower seeds are readily available in the shell. Taking the time to open each shell individually completely changes your eating pattern with this tasty snack. Remember to read the ingredient list. The only ingredients should be nuts and perhaps salt. Avoid nuts that are coated with anything else. Some nuts come coated with sugar. Many dry-roasted nuts come coated with MSG and other items.

While we are talking about nuts, I should mention nut butters. Real nut butters are nutritionally equal to real nuts. Unfortunately, food processors learned long ago that if they took the peanut oil out of peanuts, they could sell it separately at a high price. They then could grind the peanut residue and mix it with cheap cottonseed or soybean oil, add sugar, and market this imitation product to your children. This has been going on for so long you may have never tasted real peanut butter. Fortunately, there is a movement back to the real thing, with at least one national brand selling real peanut butter. Even better, a few large markets and gourmet shops use a machine that grinds fresh roasted peanuts into pure peanut butter while you watch. There are also some health food shops selling nut butter from more expensive nuts, such as almonds and cashews. Check them out and sample these interesting products.

The last item to consider in the snack department is very different. Unflavored bacon rinds are a common snack food in some places while others turn up their nose at this product. If you eat pork products, try them. They can be crushed and used as a bread crumb substitute in cooking. They can satisfy a craving for a crunchy snack and can be used as a substitute for chips for use with dips. Get them fresh. Stale bacon rinds become rancid and taste bad. Always buy the unflavored variety, which has no MSG.

Now you are ready to head to the cashier. Buying real products instead of imitation products is costly. At first, it may seem that your grocery bills are higher due to buying these more expensive products. With time, you should notice these costs go down because you lose your craving for junk food and you will be buying foods in smaller quantities. Most people find that one balances out the other. Even when it does not, after a few weeks on this diet people do not ever want to go back to the imitation foods. They feel better eating real foods that taste so much better.

During your first few visits to the grocery store, prepare for the extra time that it will take to shop. This is because you are reading label after label until you find satisfactory products. Once you become familiar with what works and what does not work, this will become easier and your shopping time will return to normal. *The one thing that will change forever will be your appreciation of real food.*

10

Eating Out and Traveling

When you are just starting your diet, the thought about eating away from home can be scary. At home you have control over your environment, but questions arise when you will have to eat away from home. Some problems are easily solved while others pose a real dilemma. This chapter deals with strategies that many different people have developed.

Questions about eating out and traveling are probably the most frequent issue that comes up as new dieters join our support groups. Fortunately, the wisdom within the group often prevails. There is generally another group member who has faced something similar and will explain how she or he did it. This chapter is a compilation of various strategies that have come from these groups. Your situation may not be exactly the same, but you may be able to glean enough from their wisdom to find the answer to your problem.

Avoid Eating Out

This is the simplest strategy of them all. It may seem rather limited, unless you ask yourself, "Do I really need to eat out on this occasion?" Many times, we choose to eat out because it seems like the simplest alternative. If you really do not need to, do not do it and you avoid any conflict.

Get to Pick the Spot

When going out with a group, it pays to be assertive. Sometimes, groups have a hard time deciding where to go and just by being assertive, you can provide an answer. At other times, you may need to be more forceful and state that you can only go if certain places are avoided. Finally, if with friends, play the diet card. Explain that you are on a restricted diet and only particular places will meet your needs.

Skip It

One dieter works in an environment where the staff orders out for pizza the same day each week. Her strategy is to fast that day every week. Because she now fasts easily, she does not feel deprived by missing a meal and not joining her colleagues.

Avoid Buffets

You may be able to pick the right foods from a buffet but it is difficult. All-you-can-eat restaurants make their money by emphasizing cheap food. That means that much of what they put out is high in carbohydrate. If they serve meat or chicken, it is likely to be a cheaper cut made tastier with MSG. An additional trap is that you may feel compelled to get your money's worth when eating at this type of restaurant. These are dangerous places for dieters and best avoided.

Ask for a Take-Home Box

Instead of waiting until the end of the meal, have a take-home container brought to you when your food comes to the table. Put the excess food into the box and just leave the part you should eat on your plate.

Split a Meal

If you are eating out with another dieter, splitting a meal is a sensible strategy. Most restaurants will go along with it.

Hold the Sides

Be sure to clearly tell your waiter or waitress that you do not want the potatoes, muffins, bread, or other items that they include as side orders with your dinner. Surprisingly, some may argue with you, so be assertive. Perhaps they think they are doing you a favor by bringing all the food you paid for.

Ask for Alternative Side Dishes

The smarter waiters and waitresses will want to cooperate with you and provide alternatives, even when they may not be listed on the menu. Let them know you would be happy to pay a small extra charge to replace the potatoes with a vegetable.

Order Eggs

Some restaurants have a twenty-four hour breakfast policy. See if you can order eggs, no matter what time of day it is. Try to order them without extra items you do not want to eat.

Ask for a Side Order

Chain restaurants may be slaves to their computer systems. They may resist accepting an order for eggs without the associated pancakes and other trappings, if it is ordered as a main course. However, the server often has an alternative of putting in an order as a side order for just the specific item you want. Ask for it.

Ask for Alternative Menus

Many restaurant chains have special alternative menus for those with particular dietary needs. These may be children's menus, senior menus, menus for people with gluten restrictions, menus for diabetics, and menus for dieters. Do not be afraid to ask about them, all they can say is no. If you are neither a senior nor a child, some servers will think you are being cheap by ordering from a special menu. Explain that you are dieting. If necessary, get your doctor to sign a small card like the one shown below. Carry it with you for argumentative servers. I provide this for dieters under my care and it seems to work. When used, dieters have received complete cooperation.

Mary Smith

is on a restricted diet for medical reasons and may be unable to consume your standard meal portions. When dining at your restaurant, your cooperation will be appreciated. Please assist by allowing her/him to order senior, children's, half or side portions when available.

Thank you for your help.

Jane Doe, M.D.

Order Appetizers

An appetizer portion may be perfect for your main course. If you are with a group, you may even get them to order multiple appetizer platters for themselves, instead of a main course. Some Spanish-style restaurants specialize in serving a variety of *tapas,* tasty Mediterranean appetizer dishes.

Throw Away the Bun

At a fast-food chain, you may be forced to order a small salad and small burger. Take it and toss out the bun. Many people have done it before you. At a conference where they serve box lunches, carrying a plastic fork can be handy for eating the contents of the sandwiches.

Order Salads

Many restaurants feature Chef's salad and Cobb's salad. These are often reasonable choices except for the portion sizes. Split them or put half into a take-out container.

Ask for a Half-Size

Some restaurants have half-size salads available but do not list them prominently. Ask if they do.

Hold the Croutons

Let your server know what you do not want on your salad in advance rather than have to pick things out once the salad has been brought to you.

Ask for Olive Oil

Do not take a chance on their pre-mixed salad dressing. Ask for oil and vinegar, but make it clear you do not want the house pre-mixed version. Some restaurants normally have this option available, but all restaurants have some sort of oil in the kitchen that they can bring to you.

Order Bleu Cheese Dressing

If you must use their dressing, bleu cheese is often the best choice.

Carry your own Salad Dressing

This is more difficult for a man but many women have told me that they take a small container with their homemade salad dressing in their handbag. They ask for their salad without dressing and explain that they have a need for their own dressing. According to them, no one has ever objected.

Carry Nuts and Cheese

This is a great travel strategy that may enable you to skip stopping at airport and roadside restaurants. Bags of nuts are also handy in a hotel room or at a conference where you cannot eat their lunch.

Leave the Shells on Hard-Boiled Eggs

Hard-boiled eggs that have been chilled in your refrigerator and with the shell still intact usually keep well when traveling.

116

Stay with Friends or Relatives

If you have a choice of staying in a home-like environment where you can have refrigerator privileges, this may be easier then staying at a hotel. Be sure that your host understands and will be supportive.

Do Not Stay with Friends or Relatives

Sometimes, it is easier to do just the opposite. If you plan a trip to visit family but are afraid that they will not be cooperative, staying elsewhere may be the best strategy for you. When making this decision, you know your family better than anyone else.

Stay at a Hotel with a Refrigerator

An in-room refrigerator is handy and allows you to pick up a few items, such as real cream and cheese cubes and store them in your room.

Stay at a Hotel with a Hot Breakfast

Many hotels include a breakfast with the price of a room, but it is often a high-carbohydrate Continental breakfast with few choices. However, some hotels include a hot breakfast, usually featuring items such as eggs and breakfast meats. Even if you ordinarily skip breakfast at home, this may help you get through your day's events without being frustrated when a sensible lunch is difficult to obtain.

Walk

Your diet and your activity level are often disrupted by travel. If you are some place that allows you to safely walk about, consider doing some extra walking while staying at your hotel.

Compromise on Half and Half

If you drink coffee when you are out, the "cream" they bring you is either half-and-half or that dreaded high-carbohydrate concoction called *creamer*. Although half-and-half is not recommended for home use, it is a reasonable compromise when away from home. You may want to carry some of those little tubs of half-and-half with you. They require no refrigeration and are useful in hotels which supply sugary powdered creamer for those in-room coffee makers.

Check Out Restaurants Online

Knowing what is nearby and what their menus are before you arrive in a strange city can take away some of your concerns. If you are at a conference and going out with a group for dinner, knowing the choices gives you the upper-hand in picking a sensible restaurant.

Offer to Cook for Your Host

When staying with family see if you can arrange to be the cook during the visit. This allows you to be sure that appropriate dishes will be available to you.

Plan Ahead

The anticipation of coping with travel produces unneeded anxiety. Whatever strategy you select, the act of planning ahead is helpful in relieving that stress.

Enjoy Yourself

Most dieters are nervous when they return from a trip. They are certain that they did something so horrible that they have gained weight. They are usually wrong and have either held steady or continued to lose weight during their travels. There will be times that you will do things you would not do on your diet at home. Allow yourself the freedom to be human. Just do not do anything really stupid. *And even if you do, remember that you can go back to the initiation phase of the diet and get back on track.*

If you are on a vacation, try to enjoy yourself without obsessing about the diet that you are following.

You will handle it better than you anticipate!

11

Finding the Slimmer You

Losing weight means different things to different people. One person might lose thirty pounds and be pleased with it. Another person may lose one hundred and thirty pounds and have his life totally changed. Being overweight is more than just a question of diet and exercise. There are also tie-ins to significant emotional issues. Whole books have been written about the emotional burden of being overweight; yet, diet books often gloss over this issue.

Renewing Hope

No overweight person ever wanted to be that way. The people who have come to see me have all tried many other methods and at many different times in their life. They are the survivors. Something made them decide to try one last time, one more time, and try something different. Often it was seeing a friend or acquaintance successfully lose weight they had been unable to do before. That gave them the one tool that every dieter needs, *hope*.

<u>Hope</u> *is a Necessary Tool when Dieting.*

Accepting Success

Unfortunately, many dieters have held that hope before, only to have it dashed by an ineffective diet. Surgery, pills, exercise plans all claim to hold the answer to a cure.

When these do not work, the victim is blamed. In most cases, it is the victim blaming herself. She develops an attitude that she is born to be fat. At that point, she may give up on herself. She may accept a stereotype. You know them. *The jolly fat lady. The fat but tough lady. The sexy fat lady.* Men, too, accept similar stereotypes. *Stout. Good old boy.*

Accepting these stereotypes is one defense against what we may feel is a self-failure. If we accept a false belief that we are incapable of losing weight, then we do not have to try anymore, only to fail once again. Dashed hopes from repeated failure are painful. Even a person who only needs to lose twenty pounds may feel this. A person who needs to lose sixty or eighty pounds often feels inadequate. One person may put this inadequacy in a compartment. She may feel inadequate about her physique but emphasize her other qualities. Another person may have this feeling of failure extend to other parts of his life. Unfortunately, the world can be unkind. Jokes, ridicule, job discrimination, and other negative events make overweight persons feel that they are less worthy than others.

As you successfully lose weight on this diet, you should be pleased. However, some people will be pleased and confused at the same time. If you have struggled with failure for many years, you may be confused by success. It is not you. It is not who you are supposed to be. It will not work. You are waiting for the other shoe to drop.

Learning to accept the slim you hidden under that extra fat is easier said than done. You need to get your mind around your victory.

Accept Good Things that are Happening to You.

Celebrate Success

Chart your weight-loss. Celebrate every victory. Everyone has little milestones, things they could not do before that they find they can do with weight loss. These will be different for every individual but meaningful for everyone. What these milestones are depends on who you are and how much you have to lose. Some examples have been the following:

- Painting your toenails when you have not been able to reach them
- Wearing your teenage daughter's jeans
- Sitting comfortably in an airline seat
- Crossing your legs comfortably
- Going up and down stairs without being short of breath
- Buying clothes in the regular department

This list could go on, but you get the idea. There will be some point where you find yourself doing something you were not able to do before dieting. This will occur long before you reach any final goal. The experience will be very satisfying because it shows you are on the road that you always hoped you could be on.

Milestones Reinforce Your Belief in Success.

Be Sensible about Activity

Reasonable exercise is part of any weight-loss program. It is over-estimated in its ability to take off pounds but under-estimated in its ability to improve your health and self-esteem. You may have to start out very slowly. Water exercises, yoga, and Tai-Chi are some methods which can increase your range of motion without being too strenuous. Gradually, you can increase your activity. Hippocrates had a

simple suggestion *"Do things with those younger than yourself."*
That is always a good method for increasing your activity level.
Activity can Make You Feel Better About Yourself.

Dreams may be Doable

I always use the word *dream* in questioning people
about their goals. People often come in hoping to lose twenty
pounds, because they do not think they are capable of losing
what they really want to lose. That is why I ask what their
dream weight is. That might be what they weighed on their
wedding day or at their high school graduation. They have
given up hope of reaching it again. For many people, that
dream weight may still be a realistic goal, but they had given up
on themselves. Now, once they see that they can successfully
lose weight they regain the ability to dream.

Allow Yourself to Beleive that Dreams can be Realistic.

Look Your Best

For some people, this is frightening. Some people are
afraid that looking good will bring unwanted advances from
others. Others may be reminded of attractive but shallow
people who they know. Some may be scared that their good
looks will frighten an insecure spouse. Some people just do not
want to be noticed.

Look Good, You Deserve It.

You Can Win at Many Things

If your self-image about your weight extended to other
parts of your life, changing your weight can open doors for you.

These doors were not locked by others, but by you, yourself. Losing weight, getting a new wardrobe and a new hairstyle to go with the new look can be just the right steps for some. Going back to school, applying for a better job, reaching out for new relationships are all possible next steps.

Expand Your Horizons.

Do Not be Alone

Are you doing this all on your own? If you can find support, you will do better. This is not a new idea. Call them support groups or diet clubs, they go back over a century. During the time it takes you to diet, many things can happen. You can have good and bad days. Some of these will be related to diet, others will be completely unrelated events but ones that can lead you to destructive emotional eating. Having others involved can and does help. There are also negative people around you, who may do things to sabotage your dieting. Having a support group is one defense against these negative folks.

Accept the Support and Help of Others.

Successful Dieters Can Help Each Other

What kind of support group do you need? For most people, any type of diet support group will work as long as it is based on honesty and sincerity. It may be a circle of friends who decide to begin dieting together. It may be a group at your workplace or your place of worship. *It should not be a commercial group selling diet products*.

There are two nonprofit groups that have helped people with weight problems for half a century. These are

Overeaters Anonymous and TOPS. These groups have helped many thousands of women and men. They have different approaches to the problem, with Overeaters Anonymous focusing more on the emotional issues of being overweight and TOPS dealing more with the mechanical issue of dieting. If you need further support, both can be a resource. If you go to such a group, seek out the people who have been successful.
Stick with the Winners.

Check their websites to find a group near you

Overeaters Anonymous
WWW.OA.ORG

TOPS
WWW.TOPS.ORG

Find Support Right Around You

There is an old story about a sailing ship that was stuck because of calm winds. Its crew and passengers were running out of drinking water. Seeing a steamship come into view, they signaled for water. The steamship replied *"CAST DOWN YOUR BUCKET WHERE YOU ARE!"*

Although at sea, they had not realized that because they were at the mouth of a large river, the outflow meant that the very water they were sailing upon was fresh to drink. Often, you can find support from those around you. I consider these people the *real supporters*. As you lose weight, they provide you with positive feedback and acceptance. Learn to accept their help. Some people may fear disappointing these supporters and will reject their genuine help. *You cannot disappoint your real supporters because they accept you for who you are.* They are there for you during struggles you may be having.

Embrace your real supporters.
"Cast down your bucket where you are."

Good Friends Do Not Mean to Harm

You live in a world where there are many people. Do not let others hurt you while you are reshaping yourself, both literally and figuratively. There will be some around you who I call *helpful friends.* They often give you mixed messages. They probably mean no harm but . . .

Ignore Bad Messages but Accept Good Intent.

Some Folks Talk Just to Hear Themselves

There are other folks around you who can be quite harmful. Some are casual observers, who really do not care about you but still can make harmful remarks. They may be ignorant or think that they are funny. Like the last group, they too, are best ignored.

Learn to Ignore Ignorance.

Other Folks are Threatened by Your Success

Finally, there are the truly nasty ones. They bring you cookies when they know you are dieting. They criticize whatever methods of diet you are using, saying it can not be healthy for you. They tell you that you look terrible as you become slimmer. They do all these things wearing a smile and saying that they mean it in your best interest. **These people have problems of their own.** Sometimes they are overweight and resent it when someone else is successful at losing weight. They may feel that your success highlights their own failures.

Pity the Nasty Folks.
They Have Problems of Their Own

Points for Success

- *<u>Hope</u> is a necessary tool when dieting.*
- *Accept good things that are happening to you.*
- *Milestones reinforce your belief in success.*
- *Activity can make you feel better about yourself.*
- *Allow yourself to beleive that dreams can be realistic.*
- *Look good, you deserve it.*
- *Expand your horizons.*
- *Accept the support and help of others.*
- *Stick with the winners.*
- *Embrace your real supporters. "Cast down your bucket where you are."*
- *Ignore bad messages, but accept good intent.*
- *Learn to ignore ignorance.*
- *Pity the nasty folks. They have problems of their own.*

12

Leveling Off

When my patients see that they are losing weight successfully on this diet, they begin to ask questions about maintaining their loss. I answer that they will not need a "maintenance diet" because when they reach the point of leveling off, they will have developed their own individual plans for how to live their lives. As you first read this, you may wonder what this means, but after you have been losing weight for a few weeks you will understand.

This is not simply a diet; you have been changing your lifestyle. Look back at what you have already done. If you are now in the weight-loss stage, you have already taken important steps in making this change:

- Your maintenance plan began the day you cleaned your cupboards of harmful faux foods. That action was a first step in declaring your independence from foods that may harm you.

- The next step that you took was to greatly reduce your carbohydrate intake.

- As you changed the mixture of foods you were eating, you gained a better understanding of the need for balance within your diet.

- You kept close watch on your food intake, your metabolic state, and your weight. Doing this helped you learn what works for you.

- You began to feel better physically, and your energy level changed.

- As you began to lose weight, you increased your activity level in a way that was sensible for you.

- If you are working with your doctor because of issues such as high blood pressure or diabetes, you probably saw your need for medication reduced. You learned that you have the power to prevent or control disease - even when problems have already begun.

- As you learned that you were not helpless or a failure in controlling your weight, your self-esteem and outlook on life improved.

- You learned that rigid mealtimes were not required when your body had enough energy.

- You found that as your body became more efficient, your energy needs were reduced and you needed to make adjustments to your diet to maintain a steady course.

- You may have discovered sensitivities to certain foods which made you feel bad.

- You may have discovered "trigger foods" that set you off on an eating binge.

- You may have made some mistakes, but you learned from them. You developed the habit of not feeling sorry for yourself with each mistake you made. Instead, you learned to recognize what your weaknesses were, both metabolically and emotionally.

- You discovered that brief fasts are one way to reset your metabolism at times when you have gone astray.

- You may have noticed that there is more to losing weight than simply shedding fat as your body remodeled itself.

- You became optimistic about your future as you began to look, act, and feel younger.

These are accomplishments for which you can be proud. Congratulate yourself for what you have already done. This is a good time to put aside irrational fears based upon previous experiences when you may have regained weight after losing some. Re-read the list of what you have already done. You have learned to use tools that will see you through this next stage.

Some people call this "maintenance," but I prefer to think of it as leveling off. Consider a pilot who has successfully taken off in an airliner. Next, she navigates successfully to her destination. She makes some normal course corrections accurately during the journey and uses her gauges to let her know how she is doing. As the plane burns fuel, it becomes lighter and runs more efficiently. The pilot adjusts for these changes as she goes along. When the destination is in sight, she followed a specific path to come back to earth and keep the landing smooth. Because each aircraft has different characteristics and conditions vary, her landing may not be the same as another's. Once she has landed, she taxies to the terminal gate where she can shut down the engines and relax.

When you are ready to level off, you too will have successfully taken off, followed a path, made adjustments and now have your destination in sight. It is the time for you to successfully land. You have the knowledge and experience to do it, if you look back at what you have done so far.

If you stay up in the air, your journey is not complete. Leveling off is a process that takes certain steps. Like the pilot's steps, these may not be identical for everyone. Follow these general steps to guide you:

- **Do not dream of going back to your old eating habits or you will keep yourself in a never-ending pattern, flying in circles but never reaching your destination**. Albert Einstein was quoted as saying that insanity could be defined as repeating the same mistakes of the past and expecting them to come out differently. Expecting to successfully lose weight and return to the eating pattern that previously created your problem fits that definition of insanity.

- **Re-evaluate your goal.** If you had to shed a lot of weight, your body has been going through significant remodeling. You first set your goal as if the amount of muscle and bone would not change. If you had a considerable amount to lose, more change could be taking place. All that extra muscle and bone needed to carry your extra weight is no

132

longer needed and may have reduced. On the other hand, your higher activity level may have created more muscle and stronger bones in other places. If these changes are occurring, consider a re-evaluation to decide on a long-term target weight.

- **Plan a steeper flight path before leveling off.** As you begin to shift your body to a steady state, it will regain some short-term storage. When you started to diet, you rid yourself of glycogen and its associated water. That told your body to burn stored fat. As you level off, it is normal for your body to rebuild some of that glycogen. Allow yourself a few pounds for that purpose. Everyone will differ, but I suggest allowing your weight-loss diet to continue about four to six pounds below your goal. As your body rebuilds its stored short-term glycogen, this natural readjustment should level you off at your goal.

- **Stay in touch with your doctor.** This is particularly important if you were started or stopped on any medication while dieting. If he or she ordered baseline lab tests, this is a good time to recheck them.

- **Continue to avoid flavor-enhancers.** Free glutamates such as MSG have been our focus because they are overeating triggers. Continue to avoid them.

- **Continue to avoid high-sugar foods.** Today, the average American consumes about <u>twenty-five times as much sugar</u> as did Americans at the time of the American Revolution. Since you may have acquired a high-sugar taste, continue to use artificial sweeteners as long as you need them. Your body has learned to associate the sugar taste with the brief good feeling from the sugar rush.

As you continue to develop into a sugar-free person this association will weaken and with time, your body will no longer demand over-sweetened foods. If you are raising children, try not to get them hooked on the need for that sweetness. Instead, they will learn to appreciate sweet foods as the special treat that they should be.

- **Add foods gradually.** By adding foods one at a time, you can discover if you are sensitive to certain foods and learn to avoid those foods. You may have been suffering from a food sensitivity, irritable bowel syndrome or celiac disease and not even known it. Some people might feel better as their conditions respond favorably to the simpler, purer foods they are now eating. By adding foods slowly, you will be aware of reactions to particular foods.

- **Watch out for and accept your food addictions.** Some people were overweight simply because they ate too much, but others may have been changed by their overeating. Some people will have become actual food addicts, where the chemistry of certain foods triggered a cascade of both biochemical and psychological events that caused them to eat even more.

One person may decide to eat one chocolate chip cookie and be perfectly okay while another will find she has eaten the whole plate of cookies before the evening is over. She was not bad or weak-willed. Instead, she had a food addiction that was triggered by that one cookie and she should totally avoid that trigger food in the future. The person who was able to eat the cookie should not be smug about it. Although not a trigger for her, some other food might be. That is another reason to add new foods one at a time. It helps identify problem foods that create these addiction issues for you

- **Be alert to the presence of other contaminants.** There are many other substances found in our food that are currently allowed by lax government watchdogs. Some have other potential for harm but have not been banned because of incomplete scientific data, bureaucratic foot-dragging, and misleading information from the food industry. Although these may not be diet-busters, if they have the potential to harm you and your family, ask yourself if you really want them in your food.

- **Continue your activity level.** Hopefully, you have developed an exercise pattern that you really enjoy, not one you glumly dread because it is the "right thing" to do.

- **Continue to track your food intake and your weight.** Do this as closely as when you were dieting for the first few months. You will be able to spot some patterns that are danger spots for you.

- **Fast periodically, even if you do not need to lose weight.** This will help insure that the energy pathways you re-opened during this diet continue to stay open. Recently, cardiology researchers studied members of the Church of Jesus Christ of Latter-Day Saints (Mormons) and discovered that those who fast monthly for religious purposes are healthier.

- **Eat less than the government tells you to.** Most dietary guidelines the U.S. Government issues are too generous. They are set with wide safety margins to prevent malnutrition and are a very real factor in over-feeding many people with more calories than they actually need. After World War II, a remarkable thing happened. The devastation of war created food shortages throughout Europe. These shortages continued for several years until the United States intervened and provided massive aid through the Marshall Plan. While Europe was short on food, death rates fell. This phenomena has been duplicated in the laboratory time and again. Eating a little less lengthens life.

- **Plan your maintenance calories.** Since you are not going to attempt to eat as much as you did before, how much should you eat? Personalize your food intake to your needs. Start by going back and reviewing your daily logs. The records you have been keeping should tell you what your energy need is. Look for the time just before you began leveling off. Perhaps you were eating about 800 kilocalories each day but your rate of weight loss had dropped to a pound each week for several weeks. One pound weight loss each week is roughly equal to an energy deficit of about 600 kilocalories each day. Add that 600 to the 800 you were eating and that brings you to about 1,400 kilocalories per day to maintain a steady weight.

  Whatever your number is, it is more likely to be correct than the government's one-size-fits-all recommendation. As you level off, try it and see if this amount of food will keep your weight steady. Research suggests that keeping your food intake at the level that maintains your weight **and no more** is associated with good health and longevity.

- **Eat locally.** Shop at farmers' markets and grow some of your food, if you can. Even city apartment dwellers can grow small window-box and balcony gardens. Knowing who grows your food goes a long way to assuring its freshness and purity. It is also the right thing to do ecologically, since the food you eat will not have been shipped thousands of miles to get to you.

Learn about getting real food from
local farmers at
www.localharvest.org

- **Eat seasonally.** The ancient advice of Ecclesiastes is still worthwhile today. "A season is set for everything…." Today, with most of us far removed from agriculture, we forget this and demand foods out of season.

  Not so long ago we could look forward to the fall, when we could expect to eat fresh, crisp apples. There is an old religious practice of offering a special prayer of thanksgiving the first time you eat a particular fruit or vegetable each year. This simple and joyous practice expresses gratitude for reaching that season. If you visit an orchard when fruit has ripened, you will understand this. The appreciation for nature's wonders and gratitude for enjoying special foods in season simply is not the same when a New Yorker can buy a fresh apple flown in from New Zealand in the spring. Eating seasonally helps your body regulate itself and makes you appreciate the bounty available to you.

- **Eat traditionally.** Selective breeding is a powerful tool that has been used sparingly by agriculturalists for millennia. Over time, implemented slowly, it has helped the human food supply to expand and improve. Today, we see our food changing at a dizzying rate. Massive research has changed this selection process and has been quickened even further by genetic engineering. Some of these new products may prove useful but others could be dangerous.

  Time answers many such questions but today chemical companies and food processors have banded together to create foods that offer the most short-term profit for them. Whether it is turkeys bred to grotesque shapes to vary the balance of their meat, apples that grow to the portion size of a softball, or grain that produces its own internal insecticide, a few years of lab study is often inadequate to show all the potential drawbacks. Look for "heritage foods" whenever you can find them. Many small farmers are going back to these, creating a niche market not served by the giant producers.

- **Learn about your own true heritage.** Our nation is a vast melting pot. Even if your genetic roots can be traced back to a single group, it is unlikely that your food traditions are as pure. Many cultures based their traditional food choices on a combination of availability and health. Genetic traits sometimes play a powerful role in the development of food traditions.

  For example, there are cultures that turn milk into fermented kefir or yogurt. This strategy makes sense in parts of the world where lactose intolerance is common, such as Africa and the Mediterranean region. Otherwise, the dairy product would cause gas and diarrhea for those carrying this gene. However, it would not serve the same purpose in Holland or Germany, where this genetic problem is uncommon.

When you investigate traditional foods, be careful which tradition you use. For example, foods that became "traditional" during a period of deprivation or limitation are not a good choice. One example is *Indian Fry Bread.* Today, this supposedly traditional food is found at many Native American gatherings. It is not truly traditional, but instead came into use when tribes were forced from their ancestral homes and provided rations of flour and lard by the government. Look back far enough as you search your heritage for foods from good times.

- **Make exceptions for *very special occasions*.** It may be that you are attending your daughter's wedding or your grandparents' fiftieth anniversary. These are not everyday events, and you may feel that you should have a slice of a cake you would otherwise avoid. Okay, you are human and if you decide to do something like that, have a plan. Do not guilt yourself into saying "I broke my own rules so I may as well go all the way."

  Instead, be ready to adjust to compensate for going off track and enjoy the special event. Learn to consider these decisions and have a plan to quickly resume your healthy behavior. If you choose to do this, do not do it too often. It is easy to become complacent after doing this once without a problem. If you do this often, you could revert to a pattern of yo-yo dieting, constantly regaining and re-dieting in an unhealthy pattern.

- **Think about your looks wisely.** If you have been increasing activity and exercise, you may be pleasantly surprised as you tightened up. For some, stretched skin may appear less attractive and a reminder of your overweight old self. Enjoy your healthier, new-found body, even if you worry that it is not perfect. Those around you may be telling you how good you look. Accept their compliments, and do not rush to extreme measures.

  Do not try medications or make-up that promises to rid you of wrinkles. This may harm you by irritating your skin to puff it out, not a healthy state. If you are considering having a cosmetic surgeon tighten your skin to match your leaner body, wait a bit. I am not against such cosmetic surgery, so long as you make such a decision slowly and wisely. First, continue to exercise and maintain your new weight for a year or so. Be sure that the person offering to provide such cosmetic surgery is fully residency-trained and Board-Certified in Plastic Surgery. Be sure that you have a long talk with the surgeon before you decide to proceed. The best surgeons will want to be sure that you are realistic and will benefit before they agree to proceed.

- **Help others who need to lose weight.** This action is not purely altruistic. By using your personal experience to help others, you will be reinforcing your own healthy behavior. There are many ways to do this. You may be an example for your family. You may be a support system for friends who are trying to lose weight. You could form a weight-loss support group with acquaintances at your workplace or place of worship. You might attend one of the nonprofit weight-loss support groups, such as TOPS or Overeaters Anonymous. Whichever way you do it, you can feel good about helping another person while actually also helping yourself.

All of these recommendations are not a "maintenance diet" but lifestyle changes. Because of individual differences, there cannot be one fixed diet for everyone. I recommend that you use a process of finding the food mix that works best for you.

For many, this process may result in what I call a **Modified Mediterranean-style Diet** *(see the boxes beginning on the next page for further discussion).*

Start by reviewing the weight-loss diet you just completed. You should have been getting an adequate foundation of protein and fat. You may increase your protein moderately. As you begin to increase your carbohydrate intake, do so mostly in the form of vegetables, peas, and beans. Try modest amounts of fruit that is in season. If you find yourself increasing your fat intake, do so with healthy ones, such as olive oil. Try small amounts of milk or yogurt. Keep things made from grains among the last additions to your diet.

- **Use your experience with your food diary to estimate the energy you need as you vary your diet.** Remember to add foods one at a time. Give each new food a few days and watch your reaction. Foods that cause you to eat more than intended may be trigger foods and you should avoid them.

- **Foods that cause gastrointestinal distress should be noted and avoided.** If you discover some, you may have a food allergy, a food sensitivity or a disorder such as *Irritable Bowel Syndrome* or *Celiac Disease.* *Continued on page 146*

What is a Modified Mediterranean-Style Diet?

Much has been written about the health benefits of the so-called *Mediterranean Diet* in recent years, but what does it really mean? Since the diet of nations bordering the Mediterranean Sea varies widely, some nutritionists attempt to rationalize the discredited USDA food pyramid by using similar food combinations to describe Mediterranean eating habits. In fact, some of the diets they describe as supposedly representative are from poor regions that rely heavily on cheap grains. Although olive oil is synonymous with a healthy Mediterranean diet, the average consumption of olive oil can vary by a factor of ten or twenty times between different parts of the Mediterranean. To avoid confusion with these other diets, I use the term ***"Modified Mediterranean-Style Diet,"*** relying on certain features of food consumption in the Greek Isles.

The wonderful diet of that region is a result of Greek geography. The rugged terrain of the Greek Isles makes the olive tree a preferred agricultural crop and a major food source. The olive became a source of great wealth in ancient times as the Greeks exported large quantities of this healthy oil throughout the ancient world.

Today, the average consumption of olive oil per person in Greece is more than twenty times that of the average American. Looking at olive oil alone, an average Greek may consume almost a third of their energy intake from this healthy oil. In addition, the Mediterranean Sea surrounding the Greek Isles provides the wealth of fresh fish that is another important part of the Greek eating tradition. *(continued)*

Modified Mediterranean-style Diet
(continued)

In addition to the fat coming from olive oil, Greeks consume other fats from fish, nuts, meat, cheese, and other dairy products. This total of all these fats is well above the 30 percent energy recommendation from fat that heart experts talk about in the United States. Yet, Greeks have a lower level of heart disease than we do here in America. The reason is the positive benefit of a diet high in olive oil, fish, and nuts as is found in Greece.

Protein from fish, meat, and eggs is present in moderate amounts, but what about carbohydrates? Simply put, a diet with this higher percentage of healthy fat has to displace something. In this case, healthy fat replaces carbohydrates for energy intake in a way that reduces the total amount of carbohydrates eaten.

Next, what types of carbohydrates am I recommending? Mixtures of vegetables including peas and beans with limited amounts of whole grain are the healthiest carbohydrate mixture. However, people who were previously addicted to carbohydrates have to be cautious in case some of these are trigger foods for them.

Finally, allow yourself modest amounts of high sugar foods, primarily from fresh fruit in season. The very last items to cautiously sample are sweetened foods, in very small amounts. Items such as pastries covered with honey should be reserved for holidays and other festive occasions.

If you suspect such a problem, check with your doctor or a gastroenterologist. Special support groups can provide you more information on either of these and help you learn what foods to avoid. You may not have noticed the connection between eating and feeling ill before. Instead, you just felt better on a limited diet while losing weight. As you add these foods back, the difference may be noticeable.

• **If you are diabetic and were able to reduce or eliminate medication while losing weight, be careful.** Monitor your blood sugar closely and work with your doctor. See if you can identify an eating pattern that will keep you in good control with the least need for medication.

• **If maintaining a steady level of ketosis gave you a feeling of well-being and mental clarity, keep close watch on yourself and your mental state.** If you begin to notice a return to your old self, you may be sensing brain chemistry changes as you drop out of ketosis. If this occurs, you should determine how you can maintain your healthier state **without further weight-loss**. You do not want to join the ranks of those suffering from anorexia, people who starve themselves by continually dieting. If you need to deal with this issue, I can suggest three strategies, but caution you to examine each of these with your physician and only use them with his or her supervision:

    1. **Try to maintain this mental balance through periodic brief fasts.** If you attempt this, watch your weight to be sure you do not overdo it.

    2. **Follow a ketogenic diet that is <u>not</u> intended to reduce weight.** These higher-fat diets are

sometimes called Inuit or Eskimo diets, because native people of the far north traditionally ate like this. They did not have health problems until "civilization" radically changed their diets. Another group who continues to follow a high-fat diet are certain nomadic shepherds of central Asia, noted for living longer than most people elsewhere.

Such diets require you to keep your carbohydrate level as low as it was when you were losing weight but increase the energy in your diet by increasing the healthiest fats, such as olive oil, fish, foods with higher levels of omega-3 fatty acids, and omega-3 supplements. Have your physician check your lipid levels to verify that you are doing this in a way that will not cause negative changes in your cholesterol.

3. **Consider anti-depressant medication.** The changes in your brain chemistry from your weight-loss and ketosis may have helped you overcome a case of clinical depression. If getting off the weight-reduction diet triggers a return to depression and is not amenable to other strategies, work with your physician to find a medication that is right for you. Take into account the issue of some of these medications triggering significant weight-gain.

These last three strategies are not general suggestions. They are reserved for a very special situation and intended to be used *only* when working closely with a physician who understands these issues. Most people should do well with a modified Mediterranean-style diet, once they customize it to their individual needs.

Keep your old daily logs, should you ever need to get back on track. Once routine, you will no longer monitor every move. Instead, it will become a new lifestyle for you. When you have dealt with your own overweight issues and learned that you have the ability to control it, you have opened the door to a newer and healthier lifestyle.

Go and enjoy it.

13

Protecting your Family

There is ancient religious dictum that states *"If you save one life it is as if you have saved the entire world."* If every person in the world were able to save just one life, it would change the entire world. At the beginning of this book, I explained the magnitude of the obesity epidemic. It is affecting the entire world. How can you, simply a dieter, expect to change the world? The answer is that you begin one person at a time.

First of all, begin with yourself. As you become successful in your dieting, you will become an example for those around you. Family members who were reluctant to admit their own need for weight-loss can suddenly become interested. Your example can lead them to save their own life. The obesity epidemic we are facing is killing people. Anyone who you have encouraged by your example can be a life that will be saved.

You may not think of yourself as a crusader or leader on a campaign to save the world, but what about your own family? You do not have to pressure anyone. Leading by example is one of the most powerful statements that you can make. If there are other members of your family who need to lose weight, your success can be the light that guides them. I have seen this time and again when someone who is successfully losing weight announces that their spouse decided to diet along with them and is equally successful.

When you lead by example, you do not have to be confrontational. You do not have to tell someone else that they need to diet. You know from your own experience how unpleasant that can be. People who are overweight know they need to diet but do not believe that they can succeed. Your example can give them hope, just as a friend's success may have given you hope. Dieting can be infectious. When one person in a group is successful at it, other people will focus on what they did and copy them.

This is the first way you are protecting your family and others around you. Those who are already overweight will benefit from your example. There is a second important way that you can protect those you love. Although your children may not need to diet, they might be started on the path to obesity. The knowledge that you have acquired while you were dieting will serve them well.

No, those who are not yet overweight do not need to diet nor should they be in ketosis. Instead, they need to avoid the pitfalls that could lead to their obesity. You have the power to influence them and keep them off the path to being overweight.

You can start by getting the junk food out of your house. By this time, you should have an understanding of what I mean by junk food. Start with beverages. Water is the best drink you can find in your home. If your municipal water supply has problems with taste or odor, get a filter. Even a simple filter pitcher works well. If your family has become addicted to sweet-tasting soft drinks, wean them gradually. Eliminate the sugar kick that they get by switching to diet soda. Have your children drink water with their school lunch, not those little juice boxes. Make sure that candies and cakes are treats, reserved for holidays and special occasions.

Use pure meats at your table, not the broth injected type. Stay away from ready-to-eat meals that you take from the freezer and put into the microwave. Avoid MSG in all their foods. Be especially wary of canned or powdered soups. Avoid those tasty MSG-laden cans of spaghetti and ravioli aimed at youngsters. Make their breakfast more wholesome by eliminating flavored cereals and toaster pastries. Most varieties of those breakfast foods are loaded with sugar. Use real dairy products in your home, not the imitation substitutes.

You will meet less resistance to these moves than you anticipate. If your family has seen you undergo a remarkable change through your diet, they will have a better understanding when you explain why you are taking certain steps.

Those you love are not with you twenty-four hours each day. When your loved ones are away at school or work, they are in a totally different atmosphere. As you make changes at home, educate them as to why you are doing these things. Let them know what they need to avoid outside of the home. Consider packing lunches for them so that they can avoid those school lunches, which are now under the thumb of the food industry.

Once you have your family on your side, look for other places that limit your healthy choices. Think about the potluck dinners at your church or synagogue. Suggest healthier dishes to others there. Do not be a pest about it, but explain that these are steps that helped you get slim and are helping protect your family. If the community around you has seen you get slim, they will respect what you have to say.

If you have children in school, make yourself heard in your school system. School superintendents and school boards are local. They listen to parents who stand up for what is right. Do not tackle the issues under state and federal control yet.

You will learn how that the food lobby has many state and federal regulators under their thumb. This makes it difficult for local school boards to exert independence in some aspects. As an example, you might have local farmers who would be thrilled to be able to sell fresh produce to your school. Instead, the school often must buy from major food companies, shipping from thousand of miles away, because of blanket contracts and restrictions from the state.

Instead, go after shady local practices that can be controlled . Even in small communities, local school boards can be enticed by fees running into hundreds of thousands of dollars from the soft drink industry. They pay these fees to put soda machines in the schools, replacing water fountains for thirsty youngsters. Go back to water. When school budgets are tight, dangling these huge amounts in front of school superintendents trying to balance their budgets is extremely enticing. Put your foot down. Soft drink vending machines have no place in public schools. These are your children that these companies are trying to entice. Would you let a crack dealer set up shop within the halls of your schools if he gave the school board $200,000? Of course not. Yet, soft drink companies get into bidding wars to get their brands into our school systems.

Know your enemy. The battle for good food has many enemies. Some are benign in their intent but do much harm from their ignorance. Others are highly malevolent and knowingly put their business interests ahead of the public good. Many are multinational players, who could care less about the health of individuals in your community. Some of them play dirty. The boxes that follow on the next few pages contain problems explaining how these companies play dirty and why our government is inept at fighting them. Study them and be wary. If you go beyond the local level, to your state and federal legislatures, expect to see these tactics at work.

Do not be discouraged. By starting with yourself and your family, you have a solid foundation. Working from that you can change your community. The boxes that follow show some of the problems that now exist. Understanding these problems will help you fight for a safer food supply. Eventually, we may have truly pure foods and honest truth-in-labeling, but only if people like you work for it!

If you save one life,
it is as if you have saved the entire world.

Problem 1

Weakened Safety Enforcement

The original **Pure Food and Drug Act** was passed more than a century ago. It brought about radical improvement in the trust we could give to the food industry. Over the years, the effectiveness of food regulation has been eroded as lawyers for the food processors have figured out end runs against regulation after regulation. The cozy relationship of the regulators with the regulated has worsened this problem.

Until the government looks at every single food additive and demands safety testing at least as rigorous as they do for medication, we must treat the safety of food additives with great skepticism. Until the government demands clear and unequivocal labeling of food ingredients, we must be wary of anything we eat.

Problem 2

Organized Malevolence

If you have read about the malevolent acts the tobacco industry was infamous for in the past, would it surprise you that the food processing industry they now control is following the same playbook? Just as the tobacco industry spent many millions of dollars setting up phony institutes and foundations to plead their cause, so has the food industry.

Organizations exist with high-sounding names to tell us all about food safety. These organizations are funded by the food industry. Is it any wonder that they continually whitewash and distort the truth about the dangers of food additives, faux foods, and the resultant obesity epidemic!

By appearing to be concerned about the public good, these organizations can reassure naive individuals who are concerned about food issues. Do not be one of them! You can see by your own success in avoiding these faux foods that there are real issues concerning our food supply.

Problem 3

Muffling the Truth

Right now, there is a tremendous effort to muffle the truth about pure products. There is a chemical called bovine growth hormone or BGH that is given to dairy cows to increase their milk production. Many small dairy farmers would rather produce a pure product. These small dairies have been letting the public know that their dairy herds are not being given BGH. The producer of BGH fears that this will make the public aware of the practice that many large dairies use.

To stop this threat to their chemical sale, a tremendous lobbying effort is underway in state legislatures across the nation to pass laws to silence these small dairies. If passed, dairies selling chemically free milk would be banned from saying this. Even worse, the legislation drafted by the chemical company essentially bans informing the public if any product is free of anything. This legislation passed recently in the state of Pennsylvania. Fortunately, when the public became aware of this bill, public outrage caused the governor to veto it. That has not stopped the chemical producers from introducing the same restrictions in other states.

BGH is not an issue in this diet but silencing and distorting truth is. This example demonstrates how with enough money, enough lobbying, and enough lawyers, the truth about food products can be withheld from the public.

Problem 4

Lack of Federal Health Leadership

Virtually any nation you can think of has a Secretary or Minister of Health - a cabinet position leading a government department, taking responsibility for the health of that nation. This occurs in virtually any nation you can think of except for the United States of America.

We have never had a Secretary of Health. Instead, we have had a Secretary of Health and something. Health, Education, and Welfare; Health and Human Services, and so forth. We totally lack health leadership at a level that even most third-world countries enjoy. Instead, we have a lot of small, compartmentalized government departments marching to different drummers. Sometimes they have no responsibility in a particular area. At other times they have conflicting responsibility.

Yes, we have a Surgeon General. Yet, this person is a figurehead who has no authority to command our various health bureaucracies. The Surgeon General is the ranking officer of the Public Health Commissioned Corps, a leftover from the days of sailing ships where a naval medical officer boarded ships arriving in our harbor to determine whether they had to be quarantined. That is why the Surgeon General is seen in a naval outfit. Many employees in the federal health bureaucracy are members of this Commissioned Corps, allowing them to receive benefits that equal those of military officers. The

continued

Surgeon General does not command them in their daily activities. Instead, they report to whatever branch of the bureaucracy they are assigned.

The Surgeon General is always a physician, although quite a few have been physicians who had no qualifications or training in public health. This political appointee sits at a level many layers below the Secretary of Health and Human Services in the organizational chart.

Is it any wonder that the federal government's efforts

Problem 5

Handcuffed State Health Leadership

Once, individual state health departments provided important leadership in this country. Today, health leadership within states varies widely. Although state health departments often have tremendous legal authority to protect their citizens, the federal government has handcuffed them. Restricted federal funds form a significant share of a state health department's budget. All the other things that they would like to do receive little money. For practical purposes, most state health departments find their hands tied when they want to speak out about something that is not a federal priority.

Food companies take advantage of this weakness. Whenever food companies see a state take the initiative in health matters, they argue the case for federal jurisdiction. An example is when states want to give additional package information or otherwise restrict a product. Few states feel they have the resources to battle this issue.

Problem 6

Whitewashing Dangerous Problems

The food industry knows that a consumer revolt can be a powerful force to initiate effective regulation. Therefore, they have embarked on a misinformation campaign, designed to placate the public into believing that there are no dangers from food additives.

One method that they use to do this is to plant articles in well-read magazines and newspapers that imply that these additives are both natural and harmless. As an example, when you see a food article that talks about dangerous additives as *"not having been conclusively proven to do any harm except in sensitive individuals"* that is lawyer-speak. It is intended to confuse you into believing that a substance was proven harmless. In fact, many of these additives entered our food chain without any form of testing. Others have been tested by antiquated standards that were originally intended only to keep substances such as arsenic out of our food.

This does not stop these planted pieces from appearing in important and well-read publications. They are a product of a well thought out public relations campaign on the part of the food processing and chemical industry. They are appearing more often today, as the food industry recognizes their precarious position.

This tactic is straight from the tobacco industry playbook, from when they denied cigarettes did harm!

Problem 7

Immunity from Lawsuits.

Food companies know that trial lawyers filing multi-billion dollar class action suits can be powerful adversaries. These aggressive lawyers have helped to rein in some of the nastier things in our society. It is far easier for the powerful food companies to squelch effective laws and regulation than it is to stop trial lawyers who believe they have a good case against companies with lots of money.

Although the Constitution of the United States gives citizens the right to sue when harmed, the food processing lobby would like to be above that. They think that they deserve the type of sovereign immunity given to ancient kings. They have attempted to get such immunity any way they can.

One way was to attempt to pass a federal law that would exempt food producers and purveyors from responsibility for obesity. Fortunately, this ridiculous law did not pass the U.S. Congress. However, they have been successful in another way.

A few years ago, a group of attorneys sued all the MSG producers for price-fixing. They did not sue on behalf of the food manufacturers who paid for the MSG in their packaged foods. Instead, they sued on behalf of all consumers in the United States. The theory of their suit was that the increased price of MSG led to an increased price in processed foods and so consumers should

continued

receive the benefit of this. Of course, they could not get the individual consumers, every individual living in the United States, to sign on to this. Instead, they went to the attorneys general of all of the individual states. They promised them that instead of awarding a few pennies to each individual, their state treasuries would get the money they were able to win. About three-fourths of the states agreed to this supposed windfall.

Subsequently, they drew up a negotiated agreement with the MSG producers. That agreement had these producers pay a relatively small amount of money, which was to be split up among the state treasuries and the lawyers.

The court allowed them to post a small, incomprehensible notice in national magazines telling people that they would be a party to lawsuits unless they notified the court that they were opting out of it. Therefore, any citizen who did not send a letter to the court was automatically included as a plaintiff and went along with the negotiated settlement agreed to by these attorneys. Their proposed settlement stated that **you could never sue the MSG companies for anything else**, not just things related to the supposed MSG price-fixing.

Would a trial attorney have tried to sue an MSG maker on behalf of anyone unknowingly included in that proposed settlement? Was this a tricky way to try to gain immunity from lawsuits for the physical harm done to innocent people? What do you think?

Problem 8

Stacking the Deck

Today, responsibility for food safety is split among government agencies, primarily the Food and Drug Administration (FDA) and the Department of Agriculture (USDA). Recent events have shown that these agencies may not get out into the field to inspect the processors they are supposedly regulating. In addition, they accept food companies at their word, even when the food processors buy chemicals from faceless foreign suppliers.

Food safety has always been a poor stepchild at the FDA. Many additives have been deemed safe simply because they have been around for many years. The food processing industry is happy to draft the regulations for them and tell them what to do. When the FDA needs expert advice about a food additive, to whom do they turn: people with numerous financial ties to the food industry, scientists who provide consultation to the food processors and universities with contracts from these same food companies.

14

Meal Plans and Recipes

This chapter offers practical meal plans and recipes for starting your diet. As you become accustomed to the 60-40-10 plan of this diet, you will find yourself varying what you eat and becoming more creative. However, many people asked me for a practical starting plan, which this represents. As you review the meal plans, remember their use is optional. If there are foods you cannot or will not eat on a particular day, skip them. Substitute the menu for another day or another meal.

The first section includes meal plans for a full week. Some of the food items are special recipes found at the beginning of the recipe section that follows. These meal plans are a starting point and only approximate the 60-40-10 plan. As you select menu items from them, you will still need to use your daily log to check your totals. Each recipe is in a format giving approximate nutritional totals, There are additional recipes for you to use that are not in the first seven days of the meal plan. In addition, more recipes will be available at our website www.HippocraticDiet.com and soon will be available in our cookbook. Some of these recipes are ones we developed while others have been developed and submitted by users of this diet. Some of these submitted recipes were based upon older recipes, which they adapted to the requirements of this diet. I am grateful to all those who have submitted recipes.

If you have the time, you should recheck recipes that you use, since caloric values can vary with different brands of ingredients. Because of such differences as well as variations in cooking methods, all nutritional values should be treated as estimates and exact values may vary.

Be especially wary of low-carbohydrate recipes found on the Internet. Although there are many useful recipes to be found, many contain serious errors. Some supposedly low-carb recipes from the Internet could interrupt your weight-loss progress.

Following the recipe section, there are planning sheets for you to use to analyze other recipes that you may find or to create your own recipes. If you develop recipes you enjoy, share them with others. I invite you to submit them at www.HippocraticDiet.com for such sharing or for inclusion in future editions of this book and cookbooks.

Monday

Breakfast

- Coffee with real cream and non-calorie sweetener
- One fluffy egg omelet *(see recipe)*
- One thick *(or 2 regular)* strip*(s)* sugar-free bacon

Lunch

- Small lettuce salad with two grape tomatoes
- Shredded cheese
- Olive oil dressing
- Water or diet soda

Dinner

- Three-to-four ounce steak
- Broccoli with melted cheese
- Water or diet soda

Optional snack

- One-half ounce cashews

Tuesday

Breakfast

- Coffee with real cream and non-calorie sweetener
- One fried egg
- One MSG-free sausage patty

Lunch

- Small lettuce salad with two grape tomatoes
- Sliced cooked chicken *(about an ounce)*
- Bleu cheese dressing *(see recipe)*
- Water or diet soda

Dinner

- Three to four ounce salmon portion
- Small lettuce salad with two grape tomatoes, shredded cheese ,and olive oil dressing
- Water or diet soda

Optional snack

- One ounce cheese cubes

Wednesday

Breakfast

- Homemade hot chocolate *(see recipe)*
- One scrambled egg
- One MSG-free sausage link

Lunch

- MSG-free tuna salad on a bed of lettuce
- "Free lemonade" *(see recipe),* water, or diet soda

Dinner

- Three to four ounce pork chop with optional homemade barbecue sauce *(see recipe)*
- Small lettuce salad with two grape tomatoes, shredded cheese, and bleu cheese dressing *(see recipe)*
- Water or diet soda

Optional snack

- One-half ounce peanuts

Thursday

Breakfast

- Coffee with real cream and non-calorie sweetener
- One scrambled egg mixed with one ounce cooked or smoked salmon

Lunch

- Small portion of mixed greens topped with smoked kippers
- Olive oil dressing
- Water or diet soda

Dinner

- Hearty chicken stew *(see recipe)*
- Small lettuce salad with two grape tomatoes, shredded cheese, and olive oil dressing
- Water or diet soda

Optional snack

- One ounce olives

Friday

Breakfast

- Coffee with real cream and non-calorie sweetener
- One fluffy egg omelet *(see recipe)*
- One thick *(or 2 regular)* strip*(s)* sugar-free bacon

Lunch

- Small lettuce salad with two grape tomatoes
- Sliced cooked chicken *(about an ounce)*
- Bleu cheese dressing *(see recipe)*
- Water or diet soda

Dinner

- Three-to-four ounces chicken topped with homemade mole sauce *(see recipe)*
- Small lettuce salad with olive oil dressing
- Water or diet soda

Optional snack

- Sugar-free Jell-O™ topped with homemade whipped cream *(see recipe)*

Saturday

Breakfast

- Coffee with real cream and non-calorie sweetener
- One scrambled egg
- One thick *(or 2 regular)* strip*(s)* sugar-free bacon

Lunch

- Small lettuce salad with two grape tomatoes
- Sliced cooked chicken *(about an ounce)*
- Bleu cheese dressing *(see recipe)*
- Water or diet soda

Dinner

- Four ounce portion lamb breast
- Lightly steamed asparagus with creamy curry sauce *(see recipe)*
- Water or diet soda

Optional snack

- Real cream soda *(see recipe)*

Sunday

Breakfast

- Coffee with real cream and non-calorie sweetener
- One fluffy egg omelet *(see recipe)*
- One MSG-free sausage link

Lunch

- Small lettuce salad topped with sesame oil
- Hearty chicken stew *(see recipe)*
- Water or diet soda

Dinner

- Three-to-four ounce portion of salmon
- Small lettuce salad with two grape tomatoes, shredded cheese, and feta cheese dressing *(see recipe)*
- Water or diet soda

Optional snack

- One ounce olives

Fluffy Egg Omelet

Nutritionally, this is the same as an omelet made in the normal way but once you try it, you will appreciate its flavor, texture, and size. Using a single egg, it provides about the same size portion as an ordinary two egg omelet. If you are not used to separating eggs, buy a simple egg separator at a kitchen or housewares store.

<u>*Ingredients*</u>	<u>*Amount*</u>
Large egg	1
Heavy cream	1 teaspoon
Extra-virgin olive oil (or butter)	1 teaspoon
Salt, pepper, or spice	to taste

Instructions: Separate the egg white from the yolk. Using an electric mixer or a hand whisk, beat the egg white until it is very frothy and increased in volume. Heat the olive oil (or butter) in a frying pan. Lightly blend the egg yolk and spices into the frothy egg white. Pour the mixture into the heated frying pan. Cook until done, flipping or covering to be sure that the top is done.

If you are cooking for several people, be sure to use a large pan. This recipe produces a thick, fluffy omelet. The air you whisked in will insulate the top of the omelet from the cooking heat unless you use a large pan to allow the mixture to spread out.

Energy	127	**calories**
Fat	11	**grams**
Protein	6	**grams**
Carbohydrate	1	**gram**

170

Chunky Bleu or Feta Cheese Dressing

Use this as a salad dressing, a sauce to top meat, fish and vegetables or as a dip for celery.

<u>Ingredients</u>	<u>Amount</u>
Crumpled bleu cheese or feta cheese	¼ cup
Real mayonnaise	½ cup
Real sour cream	1 cup
Hot sauce *(optional)*	A few drops, to taste

Instructions: Mix ingredients. Refrigerate unused portion.

Serving Size: About 2 tablespoons

Energy	**62 calories**
Fat	**6 grams**
Protein	**1 gram**
Carbohydrate	**1 gram**

Hot Chocolate

Use this recipe when you need a chocolate lift or to warm yourself on a dreary winter day. You also may refrigerate it to serve cold, either by itself or mixed with club soda.

Ingredients	*Amount*
100% Cocoa powder	1 teaspoon
Heavy cream	1 tablespoon
Non-calorie sweetener	to taste
Hot water	to fill cup

Instructions: Pour hot to boiling water over cocoa powder and stir until dissolved. Add cream, sweeten to taste and stir.

Energy	**65**	**calories**
Fat	**5½**	**grams**
Protein	**1**	**grams**
Carbohydrate	**3**	**grams**

Free Lemonade

This is a strategy to cope with problems when eating out, but it also works at home. When eating out, the only non-calorie beverage choices are often either water or something containing caffeine. If you do not want to have caffeine with your meal, too bad. Here is a way to fight back. It is free of both sugar and caffeine, as well as free-of-charge.

Ingredients	*Amount*
Water	1 glass
Lemon	1 slice
Non-calorie sweetener	to taste

Instructions: When eating out, ask for a slice of lemon in your water. Squeeze the lemon into you glass and use non-calorie sweetener to taste. If you tip the waitress a little more for her trouble, you still save money compared to a soft drink. At home, try using concentrated lemon or lime juice.

Energy	**0 calories**
Fat	**0 grams**
Protein	**0 grams**
Carbohydrate	**0 grams**

Barbecue and Meat Sauce

This is a terrific sauce for cooking meat and as a base for other sauces. It is calorie-free and can be made up in advance and stored. The key ingredient is chipotle sauce, a thick brown sauce made from smoked chili peppers. It can be found in the Mexican food section of many supermarkets and specialty stores.

Ingredients	*Amount*
Chipotle sauce	All quantities to taste
Ground cinnamon	All quantities to taste
Non-calorie liquid sweetener	All quantities to taste
Fresh or bottled lemon juice	All quantities to taste

Instructions: Mix ingredients together until completely blended. Quantities can be varied to your taste. Brush on meat or chicken before cooking.

Energy	**0 calories**
Fat	**0 grams**
Protein	**0 grams**
Carbohydrate	**0 grams**

Chicken Mole

Mole, pronounced **mo-lay**, is a Mexican dish which has many regional variations. It contains chocolate, ground nuts, chili pepper, other spices and sweetener. This recipe does not claim authenticity but it is tasty. Vary it as you like. It works well with other dishes besides chicken, too.

Ingredients:	Amount:
Chicken breast	½ portion, about 4 oz.
Olive oil	2 tablespoons
100% Cocoa powder	1 teaspoon
Cinnamon	½ teaspoon, to taste
Liquid non-calorie sweetener	1 teaspoon, to taste
Hot pepper sauce	½ teaspoon, to taste
Natural peanut butter	1 teaspoon, to taste
Ground red pepper	½ teaspoon, to taste

Instructions: Cook chicken by sautéing it in oil in a frying pan. Lower heat to simmer and mix in other ingredients. Stir to mix as peanut butter softens. Add a little water or MSG-free chicken broth to thin, if needed. Cover and simmer for a few minutes to allow flavors to mix. Add other ingredients, such as sliced mushrooms, if desired. You may also want to try this as a meat or chicken stir-fry, featuring cut-up leftovers and vegetables.

Energy	**178 calories**	
Fat	**18 grams**	
Protein	**27 grams**	
Carbohydrate	**2 net carbs* grams**	* see page 94

Hearty Chicken Stew

This is too thick and rich to call chicken soup. Stew is a much better description for this hearty main course. It bears no resemblance to those MSG-laden canned broths, but might resemble something recognizable by your great-grandparents.

Ingredients *(for 4 servings)*   **Amount**

Chicken leg quarter	1 (about 1 lb)
Water	10 cups
Celery	2 stalks
Carrots	2
Old Bay™ seasoning* or celery salt or celery seed	to taste
Salt and pepper	to taste
Onion (optional)	to taste
Mushroom stems and pieces (optional)	1 small (4 oz) can or use fresh mushrooms

Instructions: Use a large pot or an electric crock-pot or slow cooker. Remove any attached organs from the chicken but leave the skin and fat on. Cut the celery and carrots into about ½ inch long pieces. Place all ingredients but the mushrooms into the pot and bring it to a boil. Reduce heat to a simmer and cover loosely. Allow to simmer several hours. If you are using a crock-pot, it is fine to leave it on all day or overnight on a low setting. Cook until the meat is literally falling off the bones.

continued on the next page

Allow it to cool enough to safely handle. Use a strainer, colander or ladle to separate the solids from the broth and then carefully pick out and discard all the bones. Take out all the skin and fat and about half of the meat, place it in an electric blender or food processor and purée it. Return all ingredients to the pot, add the mushrooms, bring it back to a boil and let it cook, uncovered until you are ready to serve. For a thick and hearty stew, this should reduce to a volume of about 4 cups.

If you want to serve this as a lighter soup, begin with more water or do not reduce it quite as much. You may also want to save some of the clear broth as a base for other recipes which call for MSG-free chicken broth.

Energy *(per serving)* **257** **calories**

Fat **17** **grams**

Protein **20** **grams**

Carbohydrate **5** **grams**

*When shopping for Old Bay™ read the ingredients list. Buy the original formula, without added MSG .

Real Whipped Cream

Many people have forgotten what real whipped cream is. Once you try this, you will never go back to the artificial stuff. Have it plain or on Sugar-Free Jell-O.™

Ingredients	*Amount*
Heavy whipping cream	2 tablespoons
Liquid artificial sweetener	To taste

Instructions: Place cream and sweetener in a cool, deep bowl. Using an electric mixer with cool beaters, whip it until it doubles in size and thickens. Store any unused amounts in a closed refrigerator container.

	Alone	**With Jell-O™**
Energy	90 calories	94 calories
Fat	10 grams	10 grams
Protein	0 grams	1 gram
Carbohydrate	0 grams	0 grams

Note: Use the Sugar-Free Jell-O™ that you mix yourself. The pre-mixed cups have added carbohydrates.

Creamy Curry Sauce

This simple sauce is a great way to balance the proportion of fat in meals, while adding taste. It goes with many foods. Try it on lightly steamed asparagus.

Ingredients	*Amount*
Real Mayonnaise	1 tablespoon
Curry Powder	about ½ teaspoon, to taste

Instructions: Mix the curry powder and mayonnaise thoroughly. Allow to stand a few minutes before using. If larger amounts are mixed, be sure to refrigerate.

Energy	**99 calories**
Fat	**11 grams**
Protein	**0 grams**
Carbohydrate	**0 grams**

Real Cream Soda

Whether you want to increase the proportion of fat in a particular meal or just have a delicious beverage, try this real cream soda.

Ingredients	*Amount*
Diet soda in a flavor such as cola, cream, or root beer	Enough to fill a glass
Heavy cream	1 tablespoon
Ice cubes	

Instructions: Place ice in the glass first, then add the cream. Next, pour in the soda. Stir briefly as it froths. Drink up and enjoy.

Energy	**45 calories**
Fat	**5 grams**
Protein	**0 grams**
Carbohydrate	**0 grams**

Creamy Chocolate Dessert

This simple recipe provides a proportioned balance of energy, while allowing you to feel smug about having a chocolate treat. It is a great addition to a light meal.

Ingredients	*Amount*
Real sour cream	2 tablespoons
100% pure cocoa powder	1 teaspoon
Non-calorie liquid sweetener	to taste

Instructions: Stir together until the chocolate is evenly distributed. Taste and stir in extra sweetener, as needed.

Energy	**65 calories**
Fat	**5 grams**
Protein	**1 grams**
Carbohydrate	**4 grams**

Denver Omelet

This uses the recipe for the basic Fluffy Egg Omelet to create a Denver Omelet. The Denver Omelet was first created by Greek immigrant restaurant owners in Denver, giving it a distinct Mediterranean heritage.

Ingredients for basic omelet	Amount
Large egg	1
Heavy cream	1 teaspoon
Extra-virgin olive oil	1 teaspoon
Salt, pepper or spice	to taste

Added ingredients

Chopped bell peppers (red, green, or mixed)	1 oz
Chopped onions	1 oz
Diced cooked ham or crumbled cooked bacon or sausage	1 oz
Hot pepper sauce	to taste

Instructions: Lightly brown the added ingredients in olive oil in the frying pan, then follow the basic Fluffy Egg Omelet recipe *(page 170)* to mix the basic ingredients and slowly stir in the egg mixture. Allow to brown on one side, then, finish by turning it over to brown on the other side. Allow additional time for thicker mixtures when using the fluffy egg recipe.

Energy	**127**	**calories**
Fat	**14**	**grams**
Protein	**14**	**grams**
Carbohydrate	**7**	**grams**

The extra ingredients increase the protein and carbohydrate of the basic omelet.

Grilled Avocado

Avocados are high in healthy monounsaturated fat. Much of the carbohydrate they contain is in the form of fiber. Tajin,™ a powdered Mexican spice, is MSG-free and contains chili peppers, dehydrated lime and salt. You may wish to add a small amount of tomato sauce or salsa to the avocado when serving.

Ingredients	*Amount*
Avocado	1/2 per portion
Olive oil	1 teaspoon
Lemon or lime juice	1 teaspoon
Tajin™ or salt and pepper	to taste

Instructions: Slice the avocado in half and remove the seed. Sprinkle oil, juice, and spice in the cavity. Place on hot grill cut side up. Heat a few minutes and serve. You may also want to try cooking this in a frying pan or under a broiler.

Energy	177 calories
Fat	17 grams
Protein	4 grams
Carbohydrate	2 *net carbs** grams

* see page 94

Great Meat Loaf
6 servings

This recipe produces a moist, delicious meat loaf. It makes six diet-size portions and leftovers can be refrigerated for later use.

Ingredients	*Amount*
Ground beef (70% / 30%)	1 lb.
Unflavored pork rinds	1 cup (about ¾ oz)
Large egg	1
Salt	to taste
Low-carb ketchup (Heinz™)	2 tablespoons
Mustard	1 teaspoon
Non-calorie brown sugar substitute (Sugar Twin™)	1 tablespoon, to taste

Instructions: Crush the pork rinds into crumbs and mix in a bowl with the meat, egg, and salt. After mixing thoroughly, place in a loaf pan. Combine brown sugar substitute, low carb ketchup and mustard and spread as a topping over the loaf. Bake about 45 to 50 minutes in a 350⁰ F oven (or until internal temperature is at least 150⁰ F). If preparing in a microwave instead, allow about 14 minutes on high before checking temperature.

Energy	230 calories
Fat	16 grams
Protein	18 grams
Carbohydrate	1½ grams

Latin-Spiced Salmon

Salmon is a food that many recommend eating once or twice a week. This is an easy recipe that brings out its natural flavor. One important ingredient is Tajin,® a powdered Mexican spice often used on fruit. It is MSG-free and contains chili peppers, dehydrated lime and salt. If you cannot find it, experiment with similar ingredients. You should be pleased with the results.

Ingredients	*Amount*
Salmon fillet *(small portion)*	About 3 oz
Olive or sesame oil	1 teaspoon
Tajin™	1 teaspoon, to taste

Instructions: Place fish in baking dish. Brush top of salmon with oil. Sprinkle spice over oil. Place in an oven preheated to 375^0F (or 325^0F for a convection oven) and cook for 15 to 20 minutes. Check to see that the fish flakes easily with a fork when it appears done.

Alternatively, this may be cooked in a frying pan over medium heat. Use extra oil in the pan and turn once when halfway cooked.

Energy	179	**calories**
Fat	11	**grams**
Protein	20	**grams**
Carbohydrate	0	**grams**

Lemon-Cheese Encrusted Tilapia

Tilapia is a light fish that develops a taste based upon how it is cooked. Since it does not contain as much fish oil as a darker fish, frying it will help balance the proportion of fat to protein. Its flavor will change radically, depending upon how it is cooked. Since tilapia fillets are very thin, this is an excellent choice for a meal that can be quickly prepared.

Ingredients	*Amount*
Tilapia fillets	1 or 2, about 4 oz.
Grated parmesan cheese	1 tablespoon
Dried lemon peel	1 teaspoon
White pepper	½ teaspoon, to taste
Salt	small dash, to taste
Sesame or olive oil (or butter)	enough to cover pan

Instructions: Grind the dried lemon peel to a powder (using a clean coffee mill or a mortar and pestle) or substitute MSG-free lemon-pepper. Mix the cheese and dry ingredients in a loose bag. Rinse the tilapia fillets and pat on a paper towel so that they are still slightly damp. Coat the fillets completely by shaking them in the bag. Heat the oil to a medium-high temperature before adding the fish. Fry for about 3 to 4 minutes until the crust is brown and crispy on one side. Then turn it over and fry it on the second side until done. Serve immediately.

Energy	232	calories
Fat	15	grams
Protein	23	grams
Carbohydrate	0	grams

Halibut with Mustard Sauce

This tasty dish goes very well with steamed asparagus. The dressing adds flavor and balances the fat-to-protein content.

Ingredients	Amount
Halibut	4 oz portion
Olive Oil	I to 2 tablespoons
Real Mayonnaise	2 tablespoons
Mustard (powder or prepared)	to taste

Instructions: Cook the halibut in oil in a frying pan or alternatively, broil the fish after brushing with oil. Mix mustard with mayonnaise and top before serving. You may want to vary this recipe by substituting the creamy curry sauce *(page 179)*for the mustard topping.

Energy	**345** calories
Fat	**25** grams
Protein	**30** grams
Carbohydrate	**0** grams

Recipe Worksheet

Recipe for _____

Number of servings _____

	Ingredient & Amount	F gm x 9	P gm x 4	C gm x 4	calories
1					
2					
3					
4					
5					
6					
7					
8					
9					
10					
	Totals per Recipe *add columns*	grams	grams	grams	calories

Divide the above line by the number of servings in this recipe.

Totals per Serving	grams	grams	grams	calories

Cooking Instructions & Comments:

Recipe Worksheet

Recipe for _____

Number of servings _____

	Ingredient & Amount	F gm x 9	P gm x 4	C gm x 4	calories
1					
2					
3					
4					
5					
6					
7					
8					
9					
10					
	Totals per Recipe *add columns*	grams	grams	grams	calories

Divide the above line by the number of servings in this recipe.

Totals per Serving				
	grams	grams	grams	calories

Cooking Instructions & Comments:

Recipe Worksheet

Recipe for _____

Number of servings _____

Ingredient & Amount	F gm x 9	P gm x 4	C gm x 4	calories
1				
2				
3				
4				
5				
6				
7				
8				
9				
10				
Totals per Recipe *add columns*	grams	grams	grams	calories

Divide the above line by the number of servings in this recipe.

Totals per Serving	grams	grams	grams	calories

Cooking Instructions & Comments:

15

Questions and Answers

This chapter will answer questions that people have asked. It is worth skimming through, as you may have similar questions.

Q. This diet sounds interesting, but I do not want to give up baked goods. I love bread and cookies. Why can't I follow this diet and still have them?

> **A.** Sorry, this diet will not be much help to you if you cannot give up those treats. The carbohydrate allowance is very low for a reason. Eating large amounts of carbohydrates found in bread and cookies will take you out of ketosis. That will cause your body to demand more sugar, and the food craving that results will make it difficult to lose weight. Dieters who worried about their love of baked goods found that they did not have the craving for them as long as they followed the diet strictly and remained in good ketosis. However, when they cheated a little, the resultant craving made them want much more. Try to stay within the carbohydrate limitation and you should see your cravings disappear.

Q. I worry that all this fat will be bad for me. I would like to try this diet but skip the salad dressing in favor of lower-fat products. I will stick to skim milk instead of cream and use other low-fat dairy products. Will that be okay?

> **A.** No, it will not. The whole point of this diet is to find the right proportion of fat, protein, and carbohydrate to keep your body at its best fat-burning state. If you skip the olive oil on your salad, you lose the benefit of the extra amount of healthy fat. In addition, if you use a typical "low-fat" salad dressing, it is likely to be loaded with sugar and MSG. The same thing goes for the dairy products with the fat removed. They will have carbohydrate calories in place of fat.
>
> If you are a person who has an intolerance for fat, that is a special case. Go back and re-read the sections where I discussed gallbladder disease. Talk to your doctor if there is any chance of gallbladder disease and use some of the special products that are designed to be digestible.

Q. If carbohydrates and MSG are so bad, why aren't the people of Asia getting fat?

> **A.** They are getting fat. The governments of China, Japan, India, and Taiwan have now recognized that obesity and the diseases it causes are wreaking havoc among their people. This is in sharp contrast to our image of malnourished Asians. Rice is a staple in the Asian diet but when poverty intervenes, quantities are kept small. Now that these nations are better off economically, their people eat more. A recent study

confirmed that obesity among Chinese women is directly related to how much rice they eat.

Q. I try to follow a low-salt diet. Is this diet low-salt?

A. First, I must ask you if you follow a low-salt diet because your doctor recommended it? If so, your actual restriction is on **sodium**, a component of **sodium** *chloride* or common table salt. If you are on a sodium-restricted diet, it may be because of heart disease, kidney disease, or high blood pressure. You can easily follow this diet. In recipes that call for salt, use the substitute you would ordinarily use, which contains *potassium chloride* instead of *sodium chloride*. Since this diet avoids *mono**sodium** glutamate (MSG)* and uses smaller portion sizes, it already contains less sodium than most diets.

>   ***However, most people do not need to follow a low-salt diet.*** If you were *not* started on sodium restriction by your doctor, you could hurt yourself by restricting salt. A few decades ago, government officials began telling everyone to restrict their salt intake. Some health care providers jumped on that bandwagon, mistakenly believing that the bureaucrats had a scientific basis for their recommendations. The medical community has finally recognized that there was no sound reason for salt restriction in healthy people. In fact, there can be some pretty important problems caused by unneeded salt restriction. These include the following:

- ***Hypothyroidism.*** About eighty years ago, health authorities in the United States realized that in many parts of the country typical diets lacked sufficient amounts of iodine. Iodine is a nutrient necessary for your thyroid to work properly. Iodized salt was introduced across the country as a necessary public health measure to reduce the number of people suffering from hypothyroidism. When government bureaucrats started pushing salt restriction thirty years ago, they forgot about the iodine issue. Today, health authorities around the world are attempting to increase iodine intake in diets by introducing or increasing iodized salt in the everyday diet; yet, in the United States we have inadvertently caused some cases of hypothyroidism by doing just the opposite. *Hypothyroidism causes weight gain and depression, among other problems*.

- *Chronic fatigue syndrome.* Chronic fatigue syndrome has become a recognized medical problem in the last several decades. About a third of the people suffering from chronic fatigue syndrome may have a low total body load of sodium. Because most of our sodium is stored in our cells, a simple blood test is not enough to tell if you are low on sodium. Instead, special tests done on a tilt-table are needed. *People suffering from chronic fatigue syndrome should avoid a sodium-restricted diet.*

- *Heat intolerance.* Before air-conditioning was common, it was standard medical advice to prescribe increased amounts of salt for people working in hot environments. Salt-tablet dispensers were located next to water fountains in athletic departments, military bases and hot factory work settings. Today, when athletes face this same dilemma, they are given sports drinks, expensive concoctions designed to replace salt. *Most of these sports drinks are loaded with sugar.*

Q. I have been told to take a calcium supplement. Is that okay?

A. Yes, extra calcium is important, particularly if you may be at risk for osteoporosis. There are many calcium supplements on the market. There are differences in cost and differences in absorption. I usually recommend a supplement that balances calcium, magnesium and zinc in a single tablet. These three important minerals can be found together in readily available over-the-counter supplements. Some also include vitamin D, which is necessary for your body to properly use calcium.

Q. What is a calorie?

A. A calorie is actually a measure of heat-energy. A kilocalorie is the amount of heat it takes to raise 1 kg of water one degree centigrade. There are actually different types of calories. The one used in nutrition is the kilocalorie, but in common use, it is just called a "calorie." What we are actually measuring in diets is a nutritional calorie or the amount of energy that your body can use from a particular item of food.

Q. Everything in your diet is pure and natural except for artificial sweetener. I would prefer not to use anything artificial, can you help?

> **A.** My reasoning for artificial sweetener is that it beats the alternative. Sugar, whether extracted from cane, beets, or corn, does more harm than any other substance in our foods. If you have spent a lifetime acquiring a taste for it, it may be tough to give up. Therefore, artificial sweeteners are generally better than the use of sugar. However, questions have been raised about aspartame in particular. The best choice is not to use any sweeteners and relearn natural taste without the added sugar. That is something to strive for in your children but can be tougher for you. I suggest that you consider the natural sweetener called *Stevia*. This is an herb, which you can even grow in your own garden. It is widely used elsewhere in the world, and is just becoming known in the United States.

Q. I am a vegetarian. Many of your recipes contain foods that I cannot eat. Is there a way for me to use this diet?

> **A.** Yes, dietary limitations, whether for reasons that are medical, religious, ethical, or simply preferetial can all be accommodated. The important principle to remember is to try to use the 60-40-10 plan. Since there are different types of vegetarianism, there is no one answer. Some people, who call themselves vegetarians may avoid only certain types of meat, while others may avoid all forms of meat and fish, and still others avoid dairy and eggs as well. The more restrictions that you

have, the more creative you must be to get your necessary nutrients. Do not forget to take your vitamin and fiber supplements. If you avoid all meats but do eat eggs or cheese, you are getting good sources of protein. If you also avoid dairy, you may need to utilize tofu as a source of protein. Be careful and avoid carbohydrates, which are often present in large amounts in the vegetarian diets. Getting your fat from healthy vegetable oils, especially olive, sesame and flaxseed should be easy. Additional vegetarian recipes will be found in the companion cookbook we expect to have available soon.

Avoid vegetable-based imitation meat substitutes, which are usually highly processed soybean products, loaded with unnatural flavors and appetite stimulants!

Q. I am diabetic. Is there any way I can use this diet?

A. Yes, but you should coordinate it closely with your primary physician or endocrinologist. Type 2 diabetics respond well to dietary control of their blood sugar. Unfortunately, since the advent of oral medication for Type 2 diabetes, less attention has been paid to strict dietary modification. When dealing with a Type 2 diabetic, I only will accept them in this program if they clearly understand the major alterations in metabolism that will take place. This means strict monitoring of their blood sugar levels, usually twice a day. It also means holding off taking medication, according to their doctor's instructions, when their blood sugar levels are normal. Continuing to take medication while on this strict a diet could easily lead to severe hypoglycemia (low blood sugar). People who are not sure of their commitment to this diet and stray from it could create severe problems for themselves under those circumstances. That is why I carefully evaluate people who are diabetic. *Be sure your physician knows and understands what you plan to do.*

Q. Is there a way to focus on my big belly?

A.   Belly fat is a special case. When you are dieting, you do not have precise control over which areas you will lose from and which you will not. Exercise is one way to help tone you up, and it may help in the shape department. However, when it comes to belly fat, special things are going on. First of all, in this obesity epidemic, waist size seem to be expanding faster than anything else and waist measurement is becoming an important way to determine how sick people are. Different parts of the body contain different types of fat and some of these have hormonal influences on our health. In turn, they themselves can be influenced by our hormone levels. *A big belly is a warning of future medical problems.*

Recent research indicates that an over-the-counter supplement called DHEA *may* help reduce belly fat. This is available at pharmacies and health-food stores but, be careful. It is a chemical that the body uses to help create testosterone, the male sex hormone. Men and women have both male and female sex hormones, but in different balances. Taking DHEA may have health benefits for some but there are others who can push their balance in the wrong direction. There are people who should never take this supplement. Some women who are overweight may suffer from excessive facial hair as well as painful and irregular periods due to an imbalance in sexual hormones associated with a condition called *Polycystic Ovary Disorder*. They definitely are not candidates for taking this supplement. **Whether this supplement will actually improve health in anyone is unknown.** *Anyone considering DHEA should discuss it with their physician first.*

Q. Why do you always suggest talking to my physician?

A. I am showing my prejudice as a physician. I know that many of you will diet on your own and do just fine, but a few people may not. I recognize that dieting is a highly personal act. Your fear of being shamed by failure may make you reluctant to announce that you are dieting, particularly if your physician has not been supportive in the past.

Yet, the best person to give you medical advice is your physician, not a salesclerk selling nutrition or diet products. In this book, as well as anyone else's book on dieting, you can only get general advice. Your unique circumstances may require more specific advice. That is why I recommend that all dieters work with their physician to set individual goals.

Do not be embarrassed. Your physician has seen many patients who fail at dieting, so plan on success and your experience will help others. My experience has been that physicians feel helpless when they see their patients fail to lose weight. Your success can be eye-opening for your doctor. A significant number of my patients are health professionals. Because of bad weight-loss information, they had experienced the same past frustration as you have. If necessary, provide your doctor a copy of this book before your appointment. *Together, you can decide if this diet is right for you, set your weight-loss goal, and monitor your progress.*

Q. I am concerned about cholesterol. Can this diet upset my efforts to control my cholesterol?

A. Surprisingly, this diet is much more likely to improve your cholesterol picture. The public has been confused by the pharmaceutical industry advertising. Cholesterol is an important risk factor but the early cholesterol medications could only lower both good and bad cholesterol together. This led to a focus on total cholesterol, not because that was the most important indicator, but because it was the only thing that these drugs could appear to improve.

Importantly, the emphasis should be on lowering *"bad"* LDL cholesterol while raising *"good"* HDL cholesterol. If you are on a cholesterol-lowering drug, continue to be monitored by your physician. I generally check cholesterol levels before people began this diet and after they have been on it for several months. Most importantly, look for the ratio of LDL to HDL. That single measure is one of the best predictors of risk.

Q. Is there anything else that you can advise regarding cholesterol?

A. Eating fish, particularly dark flesh ocean-caught fish for their omega-3 fatty acids, will help improve your cholesterol picture. If you cannot eat fish, you may want to take fish oil capsules. Omega-3 fatty acids can also be found at high levels in flaxseed oil and purslane.

The vitamin niacin is another powerful way to improve your cholesterol picture. Many doctors advise their patients to take this vitamin; however, it has to be taken the correct way. Taken correctly, many experts feel that niacin is better than the cholesterol-lowering drugs. It can lower LDL cholesterol while raising HDL cholesterol at the same time. Talk to your doctor about this option.

When niacin is taken by people who have not been told how, they will experience an itching or burning sensation, and their skin may turn bright red. Although this is harmless and it only last a few minutes, it frightens many people who vow to never try this again. The way to avoid this is to take niacin properly.

First, buy the right type of niacin. It may also say *nicotinic acid* (the chemical name for niacin) on the label. It should **not** say *niacinamide,* because that is an alternative chemical form of niacin that will not improve your cholesterol. It should **not** say *slow-release* or *flush-free.* Slow-release niacin can be extremely irritating to your liver.

Niacin typically comes in 250 mg and 500 mg sizes. Start by taking a very small dose, such as one fourth of a tablet each morning. As you become accustomed to that amount, begin to increase what you take gradually until you are taking about 1,500 mg or more each day. It also helps to take a small 81 mg aspirin tablet shortly before taking the niacin. Doing this will minimize the flushing reaction so that it will probably not bother you at all. This will give you effective help in controlling your cholesterol for pennies a day without many of the dangers of some of the cholesterol-lowering drugs. ***Once again, check with your doctor.***

Q. I started out great and lost thirty pounds in the first two months. Once I got used to the diet, it became second nature to me. I love the taste of real food. The only problem is I seem to have stopped losing weight. Some weeks I might lose half a pound and other weeks I'll lose nothing. What could be going on?

    A. You may be too comfortable. Are you still keeping your daily diary (in appendix A)? Information from your diary will help you find the answer to this question. There are two likely issues here.

        First, because you have dropped thirty pounds, it takes less energy to go through your daily activities. That means that your weight loss will slow unless you are also increasing your activity level. You may need either to adjust your daily food intake downward or to compensate through an increased activity level. ***Your body burns less energy after you have lost weight. This is not a problem, it is natural and you should plan to adjust for it.***

The second issue is very common. Most people start out keeping their daily diary. After becoming comfortable with the diet, many people slack off. They may stop measuring because they get used to doing the same thing again and again. The daily diary tells the story, but if it has not been completed, it is impossible to figure out. Go back to keeping your daily diary as meticulously as when you first began. Look at the numbers. Can you see where they may have crept upward? It is often a small item that you have become so comfortable with that you stopped measuring. That gradually creeps up and knocks you out of balance. It may be that the cream in your coffee makes the coffee taste so good you have it eight times a day. It could be that a half ounce of nuts has gradually grown to four ounces. If you have been measuring and recording faithfully, you can review your diary and the problem may jump out at you. If you have slacked off, go back to keeping your log and you should spot the problem in a few days. *Making the extra effort to keep using your daily log will save you from many problems.*

Q. Eating out has changed for me. Several times I went to restaurants that I used to frequent but felt ill after eating. What is happening?

A. There seem to be three different problems which dieters repeatedly associate with eating out. You may have experienced any or all of these.

First, there is portion size. Portions that used to be perfectly acceptable to you should now seem gargantuan. After you have been dieting, your body will begin to return to normal and not accept those oversize portions. Your memory of what you ate in the past may trick you, even when your body is sending you stop signals. Use the hint given earlier about asking for the takeout box *before* the meal begins. **When you get served that huge portion, put some of it away before you begin to eat.**

Second, there is the sugar issue. Many people report that if they eat a sugar-laden desert, their thinking gets fuzzy, they get a headache, and they feel hung-over the next day. Their brains have gotten used to working from fat energy and the sudden change to the high sugar level of the large dessert forces them out of ketosis and produces powerful chemical changes in their brains. If done suddenly, it can feel quite bad. Remember, **only in our modern world have people eaten such a large concentration of sugar on a routine basis.**

Third, there is the MSG factor. Some restaurants really douse their food in MSG. The classic "Chinese Restaurant Syndrome" was first described about forty years ago. Because you have been inundated with MSG everywhere, you may have previously built up a tolerance to some of its immediate reactions, such as the headache and dry mouth that many people experience. After you come completely off MSG for a few months, you may notice the peculiar taste and sensation when you run into it again, especially when it is present in high levels. **This can warn you which restaurants and foods to avoid in the future.**

Q. Since I started dieting, I have felt calm, clear-headed and better able to focus. What is happening?

A. This is no surprise, for many people report this same pleasant reaction. It is likely due to changes in your brain chemistry associated with ketosis. There are many ancient observations about this phenomena. Whether it is prophets in the desert or a medieval treatment for the mentally troubled, fasting has long been associated with mental change. Almost a century ago, it was recognized that these changes were associated with ketosis.

Ongoing research is looking at exactly which neurotransmitters are boosted by ketosis. These changes can be similar to those from pills, but more natural and without the side-effects. There has also been recent research into how diets high in fish oil improve mental health. Such research shows the power of diet over our mental state and may lead to radical changes in how we treat or prevent certain problems.

Unfortunately, this type of research is funded in a puny way compared to the billions spent by the drug companies looking for new pills. It is common to see overweight people who have been put on anti-depressants. Although I believe that many such connections exist, more research needs to be done to pursue these questions and provide alternatives.

Imagine the billions the drug companies might lose if something as simple as dieting could help millions of people now taking anti-depressant medications!

Q. Since I started dieting, I have lost pounds at a steady rate but clothing sizes seemed to drop in big spurts. Is this normal?

> *A.*   Yes, this is the experience of many people. As you move toward your final goal, reward yourself occasionally with new, smaller clothing, but be aware that you may continue to go down in size. Save the lavish spending until you have stabilized at your goal. Do not forget to exercise and tone up. Without that extra weight dragging you down, your posture will change and your whole physique will improve. This will also improve how you carry your clothing.

Q. I have occasionally noticed that my mouth is dry and sometimes I have a metallic taste or a sweet smell on my breath. What does this mean?

> *A.*   This is a normal chemical result of ketosis. It often is not noticeable and diminishes with time. If it is bothersome, a sugar-free hard candy or stick of gum is helpful.

Q.   My muscles seem sore after a long bike ride or run. What is happening?

> *A.*   Lengthy strenuous exercise often produces lactic acid. Ketosis can also produce acid. Usually, your system compensates for this well, but the two together may require your system to adjust more. Try dissolving half a teaspoon of bicarbonate of soda (ordinary baking soda) in a glass of water before exercise. Drinking this may provide your system the extra buffer it needs.

Q. How does alcohol fit in this diet?

> *A.* Chemically, alcohol is slightly different but for the purpose of this diet, treat it as if it were a carbohydrate. Treat a glass of wine as if it were a piece of bread. If you feel compelled to have some, perhaps to join a toast at a celebration or for a religious observance, such as communion, remember that quantity counts. A small taste will do you no harm, but a full drink can easily upset your progress on this diet.

Q. There seems to be a lot of flu going around this season. What should I do if I become ill?

> *A.* Use common sense and listen to your body. If you are ill, a weight-loss diet is of secondary importance. Do what you need to do, eat what you need to eat, and focus on recovering from your illness. You will be able to re-initiate your diet when you are over it.

Q. When can I expect to find trustworthy food in the marketplace?

> *A.* This will occur when enough consumers demand it. Today, product managers for food companies see no advantage in honest labeling and trustworthy food. Some have said to me that they do not care what they sell, so long as there is "a level playing field."
>
> These manufacturers believe that if their competitors bend the truth, they must do the same to be competitive. Unlike the past, where many family-owned companies had the sort of integrity you might

hope for, food processing companies are now cost-centers of multinational conglomerates. If they do not pull the same tricks as their competitors, they will lose market share and their managers may lose their jobs.

Without improving regulation to level the playing field, it is unlikely that the food companies will change their behavior. It is up to you, as a consumer, to demand better.

"The health of the people is really the foundation upon which all their happiness and all their powers as a state depend."

Benjamin Disraeli
Prime Minister of Great Britain, 1877

Appendix A

Tracking your Progress

Use this appendix as a diary. It is very important that you track your progress. The daily log sheets allow you to do this easily. If you write the numbers in from every recipe you follow and every food you eat, at the end of the day you will be able to easily determine how close you are to your 60-40-10 goal.

Some people prefer to start each day's log by writing 60, 40, and 10 at the top of their respective columns. They then subtract the food value for each item as the day goes on, so that at any time of the day they can see how much remains at a glance.

It is not necessary to record calories, but you may wish to do so. If you do, the numbers 9, 4, and 4 at the top of the gram columns are there as a reminder. Multiply fat grams by 9, protein grams by 4, and carbohydrate grams by 4 to determine calories.

On the same sheet, there is a place to track your ketosis and your weight. If you fill these out regularly, you will be able to see how closely you are following the diet, what dishes or restaurants keep you in ketosis and what eating patterns help you to lose weight. Remember to compare morning weights to each other, not to evening weights, which will differ.

Additional diaries are available at our website www.HippocraticDiet.com. A smaller pocket or purse size diary is also available at the website, to help you record your meals wherever you may be.

Following the diary, are two graphs. The first is a daily graph to use in the first few weeks of dieting. The second is a weekly graph. Both of them allow you to quickly glance at your progress over time. The straight line (already filled in) marks the amount of loss you would have at two pounds each week. As you watch your progress and your weight continues to fall, you will have a reminder of what you have done so far, and a tool to point out when you are dieting at your best.

The New Hippocratic Diet

Date: _____   day 1 of my diet.

New Hippocratic Diet Daily Diary			
Food Item	FAT grams *x9*	PROTEIN grams *x4*	CARBS grams *x4*	Calories
Daily Totals *add columns*	grams	grams	grams	calories

Ketosis	A.M. *negative trace small mod. large*	Weight	A.M.
	P.M. *negative trace small mod. large*		P.M.

Comments & special events:

211

Date: _____   day 2 of my diet.

New Hippocratic Diet Daily Diary			
Food Item	**FAT** grams *x9*	**PROTEIN** grams *x4*	**CARBS** grams *x4*	Calories
Daily Totals *add columns*	grams	grams	grams	calories

Ketosis	A.M. *negative trace small mod. large*	Weight	A.M.
	P.M. *negative trace small mod. large*		P.M.

Comments & special events:

212

The New Hippocratic Diet

Date: _____   day 3 of my diet.

New Hippocratic Diet Daily Diary			
Food Item	FAT grams x9	PROTEIN grams x4	CARBS grams x4	Calories
Daily Totals *add columns*	grams	grams	grams	calories

Ketosis	A.M. *negative trace small mod. large*	Weight	A.M.
	P.M. *negative trace small mod. large*		P.M.

Comments & special events:

Date: _____   day 4 of my diet.

New Hippocratic Diet Daily Diary				
Food Item	**FAT** grams *x9*	**PROTEIN** grams *x4*	**CARBS** grams *x4*	Calories
Daily Totals *add columns*	grams	grams	grams	calories

Ketosis	A.M. *negative trace small mod. large*	Weight	A.M.
	P.M. *negative trace small mod. large*		P.M.

Comments & special events:

214

The New Hippocratic Diet

Date: _____ day 5 of my diet.

New Hippocratic Diet Daily Diary				
Food Item	FAT grams x9	PROTEIN grams x4	CARBS grams x4	Calories
Daily Totals add columns	grams	grams	grams	calories

Ketosis	A.M. *negative trace small mod. large*		Weight	A.M.
	P.M. *negative trace small mod. large*			P.M.

Comments & special events:

Date: _____   day 6 of my diet.

New Hippocratic Diet Daily Diary			
Food Item	**FAT** grams *x9*	**PROTEIN** grams *x4*	**CARBS** grams *x4*	Calories
Daily Totals *add columns*				
	grams	grams	grams	calories

Ketosis	A.M. *negative trace small mod. large*	Weight	A.M.
	P.M. *negative trace small mod. large*		P.M.

Comments & special events:

The New Hippocratic Diet

Date: _____   day 7 of my diet.

New Hippocratic Diet Daily Diary			
Food Item	FAT grams *x9*	PROTEIN grams *x4*	CARBS grams *x4*	Calories
Daily Totals *add columns*	grams	grams	grams	calories

Ketosis	A.M. *negative trace small mod. large*	Weight	A.M.
	P.M. *negative trace small mod. large*		P.M.

Comments & special events:

217

Date: _____   day 8 of my diet.

New Hippocratic Diet Daily Diary				
Food Item	FAT grams x9	PROTEIN grams x4	CARBS grams x4	Calories
Daily Totals *add columns*	grams	grams	grams	calories

Ketosis	A.M. *negative trace small mod. large*	Weight	A.M.
	P.M. *negative trace small mod. large*		P.M.

Comments & special events:

218

The New Hippocratic Diet

Date: _____   day 9 of my diet.

New Hippocratic Diet Daily Diary			
Food Item	FAT grams *x9*	PROTEIN grams *x4*	CARBS grams *x4*	Calories
Daily Totals *add columns*	grams	grams	grams	calories

K **e** **t** **o** **s** **i** **s**	A.M. *negative trace small mod. large*	**W** **e** **i** **g** **h** **t**	A.M.
	P.M. *negative trace small mod. large*		P.M.

Comments & special events:

Date: _____   day 10 of my diet.

New Hippocratic Diet Daily Diary			
Food Item	**FAT** grams *x9*	**PROTEIN** grams *x4*	**CARBS** grams *x4*	Calories
Daily Totals *add columns*	grams	grams	grams	calories

Ketosis	A.M. *negative trace small mod. large*	Weight	A.M.
	P.M. *negative trace small mod. large*		P.M.

Comments & special events:

220

Date: _____ day 11 of my diet.

New Hippocratic Diet Daily Diary			
Food Item	FAT grams x9	PROTEIN grams x4	CARBS grams x4	Calories
Daily Totals *add columns*	grams	grams	grams	calories

Ketosis	A.M. *negative trace small mod. large*	Weight	A.M.
	P.M. *negative trace small mod. large*		P.M.

Comments & special events:

Date: _____   day 12 of my diet.

New Hippocratic Diet
Daily Diary

Food Item	FAT grams x9	PROTEIN grams x4	CARBS grams x4	Calories
Daily Totals *add columns*	grams	grams	grams	calories

Ketosis	A.M. *negative trace small mod. large*	Weight	A.M.
	P.M. *negative trace small mod. large*		P.M.

Comments & special events:

The New Hippocratic Diet

Date: _____   day 13 of my diet.

New Hippocratic Diet Daily Diary			
Food Item	FAT grams x9	PROTEIN grams x4	CARBS grams x4	Calories
Daily Totals add columns	grams	grams	grams	calories

Ketosis	A.M. *negative trace small mod. large*	Weight	A.M.
	P.M. *negative trace small mod. large*		P.M.

Comments & special events:

223

Date: _____   day 14 of my diet.

New Hippocratic Diet Daily Diary				
Food Item	FAT grams *x9*	PROTEIN grams *x4*	CARBS grams *x4*	Calories
Daily Totals *add columns*	grams	grams	grams	calories

Ketosis	A.M. *negative trace small mod. large*	Weight	A.M.
	P.M. *negative trace small mod. large*		P.M.

Comments & special events:

224

The New Hippocratic Diet

Date: _____   day 15 of my diet.

New Hippocratic Diet Daily Diary				
Food Item	FAT grams *x9*	PROTEIN grams *x4*	CARBS grams *x4*	Calories
Daily Totals *add columns*	grams	grams	grams	calories

Ketosis	A.M. *negative trace small mod. large*	Weight	A.M.
	P.M. *negative trace small mod. large*		P.M.

Comments & special events:

225

Date: _____   day 16 of my diet.

New Hippocratic Diet Daily Diary				
Food Item	FAT grams *x9*	PROTEIN grams *x4*	CARBS grams *x4*	Calories
Daily Totals *add columns*	grams	grams	grams	calories

K e t o s i s	A.M. *negative trace small mod. large*		Weight	A.M.
	P.M. *negative trace small mod. large*			P.M.

Comments & special events:

The New Hippocratic Diet

Date: _____ day 17 of my diet.

New Hippocratic Diet Daily Diary				
Food Item	FAT grams *x9*	PROTEIN grams *x4*	CARBS grams *x4*	Calories
Daily Totals *add columns*	grams	grams	grams	calories

Ketosis	A.M. *negative trace small mod. large*	Weight	A.M.
	P.M. *negative trace small mod. large*		P.M.

Comments & special events:

227

Date: _____   day 18 of my diet.

New Hippocratic Diet Daily Diary			
Food Item	FAT grams *x9*	PROTEIN grams *x4*	CARBS grams *x4*	Calories
Daily Totals *add columns*	grams	grams	grams	calories

Ketosis	A.M. *negative trace small mod. large*	Weight	A.M.
	P.M. *negative trace small mod. large*		P.M.

Comments & special events:

The New Hippocratic Diet

Date: _____ day 19 of my diet.

New Hippocratic Diet Daily Diary				
Food Item	FAT grams x9	PROTEIN grams x4	CARBS grams x4	Calories
Daily Totals add columns	grams	grams	grams	calories

Ketosis	A.M. *negative trace small mod. large*	Weight	A.M.
	P.M. *negative trace small mod. large*		P.M.

Comments & special events:

Date: _____   day 20 of my diet.

New Hippocratic Diet Daily Diary				
Food Item	**FAT** grams *x9*	**PROTEIN** grams *x4*	**CARBS** grams *x4*	Calories
Daily Totals *add columns*				
	grams	grams	grams	calories

Ketosis	A.M. *negative trace small mod. large*	Weight	A.M.
	P.M. *negative trace small mod. large*		P.M.

Comments & special events:

The New Hippocratic Diet

Date: _____   day 21 of my diet.

New Hippocratic Diet Daily Diary				
Food Item	FAT grams x9	PROTEIN grams x4	CARBS grams x4	Calories
Daily Totals *add columns*	grams	grams	grams	calories

Ketosis	A.M. *negative trace small mod. large*	Weight	A.M.
	P.M. *negative trace small mod. large*		P.M.

Comments & special events:

Date: _____   day 22 of my diet.

New Hippocratic Diet Daily Diary			
Food Item	**FAT** grams *x9*	**PROTEIN** grams *x4*	**CARBS** grams *x4*	Calories
Daily Totals *add columns*				
	grams	grams	grams	calories

Ketosis	A.M. *negative trace small mod. large*	Weight	A.M.
	P.M. *negative trace small mod. large*		P.M.

Comments & special events:

The New Hippocratic Diet

Date: _____   day 23 of my diet.

New Hippocratic Diet Daily Diary			
Food Item	FAT grams x9	PROTEIN grams x4	CARBS grams x4	Calories
Daily Totals *add columns*	grams	grams	grams	calories

Ketosis	A.M. *negative trace small mod. large*	Weight	A.M.
	P.M. *negative trace small mod. large*		P.M.

Comments & special events:

Date: _____   day 24 of my diet.

New Hippocratic Diet Daily Diary				
Food Item	FAT grams *x9*	PROTEIN grams *x4*	CARBS grams *x4*	Calories
Daily Totals *add columns*	grams	grams	grams	calories

Ketosis	A.M. *negative trace small mod. large*	Weight	A.M.
	P.M. *negative trace small mod. large*		P.M.

Comments & special events:

The New Hippocratic Diet

New Hippocratic Diet Daily Diary			
Food Item	FAT grams *x9*	PROTEIN grams *x4*	CARBS grams *x4*	Calories
Daily Totals *add columns*	grams	grams	grams	calories

Ketosis	A.M. *negative trace small mod. large*	Weight	A.M.
	P.M. *negative trace small mod. large*		P.M.

Comments & special events:

235

Date: _____   day 26 of my diet.

New Hippocratic Diet Daily Diary			
Food Item	FAT grams *x9*	PROTEIN grams *x4*	CARBS grams *x4*	Calories
Daily Totals *add columns*	grams	grams	grams	calories

| | A.M. *negative trace small mod.   large* | | Weight | A.M. |
| Ketosis | P.M. *negative trace small mod.   large* | | | P.M. |

Comments & special events:

236

The New Hippocratic Diet

Date: _____   day 27 of my diet.

New Hippocratic Diet Daily Diary				
Food Item	FAT grams x9	PROTEIN grams x4	CARBS grams x4	Calories
Daily Totals *add columns*	grams	grams	grams	calories

Ketosis	A.M. *negative trace small mod. large*	Weight	A.M.
	P.M. *negative trace small mod. large*		P.M.

Comments & special events:

Date: _____   day 28 of my diet.

New Hippocratic Diet Daily Diary			
Food Item	**FAT** grams *x9*	**PROTEIN** grams *x4*	**CARBS** grams *x4*	Calories
Daily Totals *add columns*	grams	grams	grams	calories

Ketosis	A.M. *negative trace small mod. large*	Weight	A.M.
	P.M. *negative trace small mod. large*		P.M.

Comments & special events:

Short-Term Loss Chart

Day of Diet

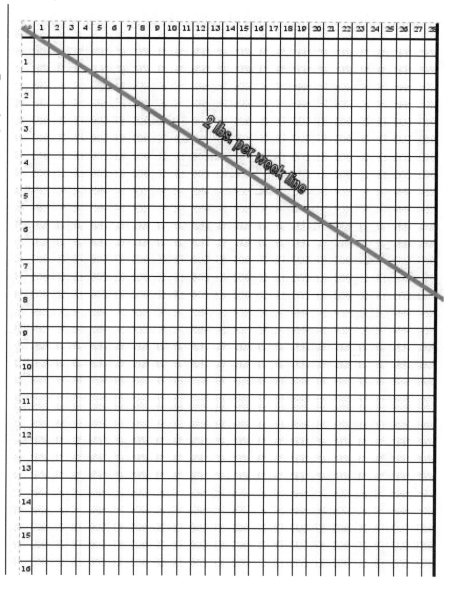

Long-Term Loss Chart

Week of Diet

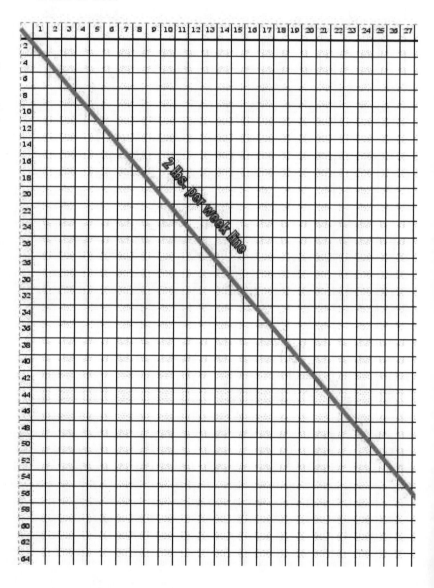

Pounds Lost

Appendix B

The Ancient Hippocratic Diet

Many questionable ideas attributed to Hippocrates go back many years. The ancient physician Galen, a Greek doctor famous for the surgical techniques he developed working for the Roman army, is partially to blame. Galen lived several hundred years after Hippocrates, but to impress the Romans, he frequently used the authority of Hippocrates in his own writings. Galen wrote in Latin, which became the language of later scholars. For many years, European understanding of Hippocrates' knowledge was limited to what Galen had said.

The Renaissance brought about tremendous change. Ancient Greek medical knowledge had been preserved but was found mostly in the original Greek or in later Arabic texts. During the golden age of Spain, Jewish and Moslem scholars provided Latin translations of ancient Greek knowledge to the Christian scholars of Western Europe. This rediscovery of ancient knowledge became an important part of the European Renaissance.

In more recent times, scholars have continued this tradition. This Hippocratic information on weight loss is not available in brief English language translations. Instead, it was a French scholar, Émile Littré, who produced the most comprehensive and respected gathering of Hippocratic works in the mid-1800s. The Hippocratic technique for weight loss or gain is found in Volume Six of the encyclopedic work of Émile Litré, *Oeuvres Complètes d'Hippocrate* published in 1849.

Major points of this Hippocratic technique, followed by my interpretations of their relevance follow:

1.   ***Dishes should be fatty and glistening from sesame oil.***

This clearly suggests increasing the proportion of fat in the diet, but emphasizes use of a healthy oil.

2.   ***The dieter should not eat bread.***

This is a suggestion to significantly lower carbohydrate intake. Bread was a primary source of carbohydrates in ancient Greece. Sugar was not the major issue at that time, since concentrated sugar extracted from cane was limited to India at that point in history.

3.   ***These changes will satisfy dieters so that they are able to eat less.***

This clearly points out the reason for the suggested changes was appetite suppression. No specific issue is made of protein, so if the amount the dieter eats is reduced, there will be a reduction in protein intake, not the increase found in some modern low-carbohydrate diets.

4.   *Eat only one meal a day.*

In ancient Greece, there was debate as to whether it was healthier to eat two or three meals each day. Therefore, I interpret this advice to mean; reduce the number of meals that you eat each day. This is consistent with reduced hunger while burning stored fat. Conversely, those who eat high carbohydrate meals must eat more frequently to deal with fluctuating sugar levels.

5.   *Work hard with younger people*

Exercise while dieting makes sense. Recent research shows, no matter what age group, younger people always exercise more. Therefore, working with those who are younger than you is a way to increase from your baseline activity level.

6.   *Sleep on a hard bed and stroll around naked as much as you can.*

This sounds unusual, and I did not include it in my recommendations for practical reasons. However, it makes perfect sense. Sleeping on a surface without bedding will usually chill you, as will walking around naked. Research has confirmed that you have a higher caloric energy need when you are a chilled. Although it makes sense, it is not very practical for most dieters.

7.   *To gain weight, a person should do just the opposite of these recommendations.*

Doing the opposite of these ancient weight-loss recommendations means that Hippocrates' suggestions to *gain* weight match what the government has told people they must do to *lose* weight.

Is it any wonder that dieters are frustrated when they followed the government's advice? Those who follow the government plan to *lose* weight are doing the very things that Hippocrates prescribed to *gain* weight. **Hippocrates' ancient work accurately predicted today's obesity epidemic.**

Appendix C

For Health Professionals

Thank you for reading this book. This supplemental section contains my opinions and experiences that I feel may be helpful to other health professionals. A number of the overweight people I have seen have themselves been health professionals, spouses of health professionals, or referrals from other practitioners. You, like many of them, may be frustrated by the increasing problems that your patients are facing due to the obesity epidemic. The recent revelations that the government-sponsored low-fat diet craze is ineffective should not be a surprise to you. When that research was published, it seemed like the small child crying out that the emperor had no clothes. The ineffectiveness of that government-sponsored low-fat fad had been obvious to most of us for some time.

Whether you see patients in a primary care setting, a subspecialty setting or another capacity, you have the ability to help to your patients on their road to recovery from the obesity epidemic. Whether you are a physician, a nurse, or a health-plan administrator, this should be important to you. It may have frustrated you at a personal level. When we can be successful ourselves, it adds considerably to the value of the advice that we give our patients. If you understand the basis for this diet and believe in it yourself, you can be invaluable in assisting your patients to lose weight.

The basis for this diet is the maintenance of a steady state of ketosis. Although ketosis in dieting is not a new concept, this plan is based upon a mathematical model for weight-loss dieting I derived from much earlier and widely accepted non-weight-loss research of others. Fasting has long been recognized as having the ability to suppress hunger. It has been almost a century since ketosis was recognized as bringing about powerful changes in the central nervous system. Pioneering work done in the 1920s demonstrated that the seizure suppression properties of a fasting state could be replicated by a diet in which proportions of food were carefully monitored. The formulas developed at that time were not intended for weight-reduction. In fact, they were intended to create a steady state of ketosis without inducing weight-loss.

My initial effort was to extend those experimentally derived formulas to encompass weight loss. This allowed me to derive an extended algorithm that was helpful in predicting which dietary mixtures could maintain a steady state of ketosis while producing weight loss. The next step was setting reasonable limits so that total dietary fat consumption was not excessive while protein consumption was adequate. This resulted in the highly effective weight-loss diet that is explained in this guide.

At the time I first developed this, nothing similar in the modern literature was accessible through Medline. I had to search earlier literature to find similar diet plans. Surprisingly, these were well accepted and well-known in their time. These led me back to even earlier work, particularly the popular but unscientific diet of William Banting (an undertaker, not to be confused with the more famous scientist) and the highly scientific diet of Wilhelm Ebstein, both in the nineteenth century.

Fortunately, contemporary quantitative nutritional analysis of their diets was available. That analysis provided sufficient data so that my algorithm could confirm that those diets were ketogenic. Ebstein's work provided the link back to Hippocrates, through the 1849 translation of Émile Littré. Although there was no quantitative nutritional analysis from the time of Hippocrates , a qualitative evaluation of the principles of that diet shows that it should be considered ketogenic and similar in its effect of producing weight-reduction.

Today, we are beginning to see a change from the thinking of the past several decades. Today, there are studies documenting the role of dietary fats in improving HDL cholesterol levels. The anti-fat hysteria is beginning to give way to a more balanced view of the role of macronutrients. Yet, after a quarter-century of bad dietary advice from the government and the media, many people are hanging on to the very behaviors that made them obese, believing that they are doing the right thing.

In this book, I attempt to instruct people in a method which has proven successful for many people previously unable to help themselves. Some were candidates for weight-loss surgery or had siblings who had undergone such surgery. Many have had their general health and their outlook on life improve tremendously. Some were able to reduce their need for medication for chronic conditions. I hope that you can be supportive of patients who wish to follow this plan. If followed, you may be surprised at their progress.

Not everyone will want to come to you for your advice and support. I have attempted throughout this book to suggest to the reader that they check with their personal physician, but some will not. Previous dieting failures make patients reluctant to announce to anyone that they intend to try again. You may have seen so many failures at weight-loss that you are skeptical that any can work and feel helpless in your inability to offer meaningful therapy. Yet, your patients can benefit tremendously from your advice and support. You can break down these barriers by keeping an open mind and letting your patients know that you support their effort to help themselves.

Consider your role as a health professional as both an advocate and a teacher to your patients. You are not unlike the general population in regard to the current obesity epidemic. If you or your staff need to work on your or their own weight issues, this is not lost on your patients. Conversely, those professionals who have successfully battled their own weight problems are examples and role models to their patients.

Combining your professional skills with support, empathy, and perhaps your personal experience will be an asset to your patients. Once you see that success is possible for those you may have given up on in the past, you may find yourself reaching out to more patients. Simple screening such as waist measurement and BMI can be handled by staff. Effective weight-loss and weight-control can become primary prevention for those you see professionally.

Should a patient come to you asking for help and advice, I suggest starting with an evaluation. I have just a few absolutes about who this diet is appropriate for. I never recommend weight-loss dieting during pregnancy. I also caution against dieting in women who are considering becoming pregnant. Nutritional needs during the first trimester are too important to take a chance on.

This book is intended for adults, although the principles of this diet are adaptable to overweight teenagers. I am aware of patients who have had their teenage children follow their parents' path in food choices.

Dieters should be reasonably mature and emotionally stable. They should be willing to give up alcoholic beverages when dieting. Although many have succeeded despite having an occasional drink for a special event, dieters who continued to use alcohol on a regular basis have had a more difficult time.

Patients who currently need monitoring of blood levels of medication should be watched more closely than others. Dietary changes will influence some of these. Those on multiple medications for hypertension also require monitoring. Rapid weight loss can result in a reduced need for medication. Such patients should be cautioned to contact you if they experience symptoms of orthostatic changes.

Patients with type 2 diabetes can be helped on this diet, but approach this with caution. Before I recommend this diet to a diabetic patient, I first determine if they are reliable enough to monitor and record their glucose levels at least twice daily. I want to be sure that their prior diabetic instruction has included withholding medications at normal or low normal levels. I review with them the danger of a medication-induced hypoglycemic episode as a result of their low dietary intake. When they are on multiple medications for diabetes, I might suggest using only Metformin for mildly elevated glucose readings.

These patients have been able to normalize their glucose readings and A1c results, using either no medication or greatly reduced medication. However, I stress to them not to be complacent and to continue testing. It is important that you coordinate this with other professionals involved, to prevent these patients from receiving conflicting advice.

Many patients report a reduction in chronic musculoskeletal problems after losing a significant amount of weight. Occasionally, a previously very heavy patient will develop problems due to muscle spasms after rapidly losing weight. This appears be musculoskeletal compensation for the effects of weight that is no longer present. This problem should be treated symptomatically, but it is better to prevent it with an exercise regimen that emphasizes range of motion. I often suggest Tai Chi to patients. An excellent Tai Chi program has been developed by the Arthritis Foundation and may be available in your area. Other good options are supervised aquatic exercise programs and yoga.

I prefer to use percentage of body fat rather than BMI in setting a weight-loss goal. You may wish to do this yourself or train your staff. Not all methods are accurate under all conditions, so I prefer to combine the use of skin-fold thickness and an electronic bio-impedance measure of body fat. Some techniques require only a single measurement and little calculation while others require up to seven measurements with complex calculations. None of these methods can be said to be totally accurate for an entire population. Therefore, I suggest that you use the best method practical in your situation and treat the results as an approximation.

Once you have determined the patient's percentage of body fat, it is a simple calculation to determine lean body mass. Working backward from lean body mass, you can determine a hypothetical ideal weight, if the patient were to lose no muscle mass while dieting. More information on doing this is available at our web site www.HippocraticDiet.com. Be sure to take the patient's weight history into account and set a mutually agreeable goal.

I usually obtain the following lab tests before patients begin to diet:

- CBC
- Chemistry panel (comprehensive)
- Lipid panel
- TSH (with reflex T4)
- C-Reactive protein
- Hemoglobin A1c

An impressive number of these patients have C-Reactive protein and A1c elevated before beginning to diet. Such abnormal results can be reinforcing for the patient, if they are presented with a frank discussion of the metabolic syndrome and the assurance that they will likely return to normal with dieting and weight-loss.

Some people will prefer to diet independently, but others will benefit from a support group. You may wish to start a professionally led support group within your own practice or simply make available facilities for a patient-led support groups. Referral to a non-commercial support group, such as Overeaters Anonymous or TOPS, may be helpful. Losing weight is often more than just a physical act. The learned helplessness resulting from unsuccessful dieting may be replaced by optimism as they regain control over this aspect of their lives. For some, the physical change is accompanied by changes in self-esteem and outlook on life. There is often a brightening of mood.

For a smaller number of patients, the brightening of mood exceeds what you would expect just from these psychological factors which accompany their weight-loss. The biochemical changes that accompany natural dieting may come into play. These patients may truly have been sugar-addicted. Although there are observations of the effect of fasting on mood going back to the ancients, there is little or no research in this area. The possibility that ketosis can accomplish this should not be ruled out. The same neurochemistry changes that are powerful enough to suppress seizure activity may also change mood.

For these few patients, I recommend that they approach maintenance very carefully. I suggest that they familiarize themselves with available information on the impact of diets high in omega-3 fatty acids and mental health. Another possibility for them may be maintaining ketosis on an Inuit-style diet, emphasizing healthy fat while monitoring serum lipids .

I try not to discuss the many potential problems attributed to the free-glutamate flavor-enhancers. Instead, I emphasize the positive aspect of removing these hidden diet-busters. Learning to look for real foods and to shop at farmers' markets can have a tremendous positive impact on your patients healthy eating patterns.

In this section, I have shared with you my opinions and experiences. I believe that the obesity epidemic can be stopped, even if it must be done one dieter at a time. Further information, and data sources for much of what I have discussed in this book, are included in the annotated bibliography that follows.

Annotated Bibliography

This annotated bibliography is being provided for those who wish further information on selected topics. There are varying types of references here, since information about the underlying forces that effect our health is as likely to be found in the financial reporting of the *Wall Street Journal,* as it is in the medical reporting of the *New England Journal of Medicine.*

Basis for this diet; development of mathematical model
This diet was developed using a mathematical model I developed as an extension to formulas for maintaining ketoses on a non-weight reduction diet. The early work on those was done in the 1920s and can be explained using the formula:

$$KR = \frac{K}{AK}$$

- Shaffer PA, *The ketogenic-antiketogenic balance in man and its significance in diabetes*, Journal of Biologic Chemistry, pp 399-441, 1922.

Research done by Woodyatt provided a mathematical basis for using this nutritional knowledge clinically. That is expressed by:

$$KR = \frac{(0.9 * f) + (0.46 * p)}{C + (0.1 * f) + (0.58 * p)}$$

- Woodyatt RT. *Objects and method of diet adjustment in diabetes*, Archives of Internal Medicine, Vol 28(2), pp 125-141, 1921.
- Talbot FB, Metcalf KM, Moriarity,ME. *A Clinical Study of Epileptic Children Treated by Ketogenic Diet*. Boston Medical & Surgical Journal (now the New England Journal of Medicine), pp 89-96, 1922.

Based upon that earlier work, I modified Woodyatt's mathematical model to take into account the differences

between maintaining ketosis on a diet in which energy
requirements are being met and one in which the goal is
weight-loss. Using that model, I derived the following formula:

$$TKR = \frac{(\ 0.1 \ast\ <e - [\ 4 \ast (\ p + c)\ ] >) + (\ 0.46 \ast\ p\ )}{c + (\ 0.011 \ast\ <e - [\ 4 \ast (\ p + c)] >) + (\ 0.58 \ast p)}$$

where:
- TKR represents total ketogenic ratio
- e represents energy needs in kilocalories
- p represents dietary protein in grams
- c represents dietary carbohydrate in grams

and when:
- energy deficit is met exclusively by the utilization of
  stored fat

- Cohen, IA. *Development of a Modified Ketogenic Ratio
  for Weight-Reduction Dieting*, Prevention 2006-Annual
  Scientific Meeting of the American College of Preventive
  Medicine, Reno, 2006.
- Cohen, IA. *A Model for Analyzing and Reversing
  Historic Dietary Trends Which Contributed to Obesity
  and Its Resultant Disease Burden*, Indian Health Service
  Annual Research Conference, Albuquerque, 2006.
- Cohen, IA. *A Method of algorithmic evaluation of
  weight-reduction diets*, (submitted for publication, 2006.
- Cohen, IA. *The obesity epidemic, metabolic syndrome
  and adult-onset diabetes: Combining a modern
  perspective and ancient answers*, University of Kansas
  Medical Center, Internal Medicine Grand Rounds, Kansas
  City 2007.
- Cohen, IA. *Using a computer model to evaluate weight-
  reduction strategies*, Kansas Public Health Association,
  Annual Conference, Topeka, 2006.

Belly fat; relationship to disease
- Jansen I, et al. *Body mass index, waist circumference, and health risk: evidence in support of current National Institutes of Health guidelines*, Archives of Internal Medicine, Vol 162 (18) pp 2074-9, 14 October 2002.
- Woo J, et al. *Is waist circumference a useful measure in predicting health outcomes in the elderly?* International Journal of Obesity and Related Metabolic Disorders, Vol 26 (10) pp1349-55, October 2002.
- Fujimoto WY et al. *Body size and shape changes and the risk of diabetes in the diabetes prevention program* Diabetes, Vol 56 (6), pp 1680-5, June 2007.
- Chen Y, et al. *Waist circumference is associated with pulmonary function in normal-weight, overweight, and obese subjects*, American Journal of Clinical Nutrition, Vol 85 (1) pp 35-9, January 2007.

Cholesterol; improvement on diet
- Hays JH et al. *Effect of a high saturated fat and no-starch diet on serum lipid subfractions in patients with documented atherosclerotic cardiovascular disease*, Mayo Clinic Proceedings, Vol 78 (11), pp 1331-6, November 2003.

Exercise; and age
- CDC. *Percentage of Adults Who Engaged in Any Leisure-Time Strengthening Activity, by Sex and Age Group --- United States, 2005*, MMWR, Weekly, September 8, 2006, Vol 55 (35), p 968, U.S. Department of Health and Human Services, 8 September 2006.

Fasting; reduction in heart disease
- McClure BS, et al. *Fasting may reduce the risk of coronary artery disease*, American Heart Association Scientific Sessions, 6 November 2007.

Government; health objectives, promoting low-fat foods
Before the government began to implement this strategy, one out of seven adult Americans were overweight. Since the government has "successfully" promoted low-fat foods, two out of three adults are now overweight.

- Public Health Service. *Promoting Health/Preventing Disease: Objectives for the Nation*, p 75, US Department of Health and Human Services, Washington, DC, 1980.
- Cohen IA. *U.S. Health Objectives for 1990: A Maryland Evaluation*, Maryland Dept. of Health & Mental Hygiene, Baltimore, 1984.

Government; public health; erosion of in the United States
- Rest KM, Halpern MH. *Politics and the Erosion of Federal Scientific Capacity: Restoring Scientific Integrity to Public Health Science*, American Journal of Public Health, Vol 97, pp1939-44, November 2007.

Government; FDA, under industry control
According to the Organic Consumers Organization, the government official who approved a Monsanto report that purported to show the safety of milk from cows treated with BGH was the same person who had written the report for Monsanto. She was reported to have been aided by other Monsanto ex-employees then working for the FDA.

- www.organicconsumers.org/monlink.cfm (accessed 15 August 2008).

Government; FDA, inability to track food-related problems
- Center for Science in the Public Interest *Emergency Regs Needed for Tracking Produce*, www.cspinet.org/new/200807031.html (accessed 15 August 2008).

Government; function of the Surgeon General
- www.surgeongeneral.gov/aboutoffice.html (accessed 18 Aug 2008).

Fat; appropriate dietary fat mixtures protect against obesity
- Wang H, et al. *Effects of dietary fat types on body fatness, leptin, and ARC leptin receptor, NPY, and AgRP mRNA expression*, American Journal Physiology, Endocrinology, Metabolism, Vol 282 (6) pp E1352-9, June 2002.

Hunger; blood sugar changes increasing appetite
- Arumugam V, et al. *A high-glycemic meal pattern elicited increased subjective appetite sensations in overweight and obese women*, Appetite, Vol 50 (1-2) pp 215-22, March-May 2008

Inuit (Eskimo) diet; and health
   Vilhjamur Stefansson was a famous Canadian Arctic explorer who lived among the native people of the north and learned their ways. He documented their diet and health and became an advocate for greater knowledge about these practices and their health benefits.
- Stefansson V. *The Fat of the Land*, Macmillan, New York 1956.

Industry; disregard for human life
   Philip Morris (now known as the Altria Group) which controls Kraft, was concerned that the Czech Republic might restrict tobacco due to concerns about health care costs. Their way of dealing with it was to commission the consulting firm of Arthur D. Little to provide a study for the Czech government showing the "beneficial" impact of tobacco. In addition to the taxes collected by the government, they pointed out the immense savings in pension and health care costs because smokers die younger!
- www.americanlegacy.org/Czech/print_czech.html (accessed 1 Nov 2001).

Industry; collaboration between food industry scientists and tobacco industry brain-chemistry experts
- Callahan P et al. *Where there's smoke, there might be food research, too*, Chicago Tribune, January 29, 2006.

www.chicagotribune.com/bussiness/chi-
0601290254jan29,0,1306987.story (accessed 30 Jan 2007)
- Manier J, Callahan P, Delroy A. *The Oreo®, Obesity and Us - Craving the Cookie*, Chicago Tribune, 21 August 2005. www.chicagotribune.com/news/specials/chi-oreo-1,1,5587986,print.story (accessed 8 Aug 2006).

Industry; fraudulent labeling
- Etter I, Kilman S. *Tyson ordered to pull Antibiotic-Free Label by June 18*, Wall Street Journal, p B9, 4 June 2008.

Industry; immunity from MSG lawsuits
The proposed settlement of the class-action MSG suit known as *Eugene Higgins v. Archer Daniels Midland Co.* dated March 20, 2006 was filed in the Second Judicial District Court of New Mexico. Although the suit was purportedly about MSG price-fixing, the proposed settlement included a "covenant not to sue," which covered any suit by consumers against the MSG producers for any reason related to MSG. The final settlement, fortunately, limited this prohibition to the price-fixing question.
- www.msgindirectsettlement.com, accessed 27 June 2006.

Industry; ingredient substitution and profitability
- Jargon J. *Food Makers Scrimp on Ingredients in an Effort to Fatten Their Profits*, Wall Street Journal, p A1, 23 August 2008.

Industry; "pro-consumer" groups front for industry
American Farmers for the Advancement and Conservation of Technology claims to "to educate, equip and empower all participants in the food chain to understand the benefits of technology and encourage consumers to demand access to high-quality, affordable food with a minimal impact on the environment." They do not mention they were organized and funded by Monsanto, maker of both recombinant bovine growth hormone and genetically engineered seeds. These are products severely restricted outside of the United States by agricultural and health authorities.

- Martin A. *Fighting on a Battlefield the Size of a Milk Label*, New York Times, 9 March 2008.

Industry; public relations campaigns
The high-fructose corn syrup producers are not sitting still for increasing consumer awareness. Instead, they have initiated a major advertising campaign to make consumers believe that they produce a healthy product.
- Vranica S. *High Fructose Corn Syrup Mixes it Up*, Wall Street Journal, 23 June 2008.

Industry; influence over the scientific community
- Campbell EG, et al. *Institutional Academic-Industry Relationships* Journal of the American Medical Association, Vol 298 pp 1779-86, 17 October 2007.

Industry; preventing small producers from identifying pure products
- Martin A. *State Revises Hormone Label for Milk* New York Times, 18 January 2008.
- Hightower J. *Monsanto fighting 'hormone-free' milk labels*, Topeka Capital-Journal, 29 December 2007.
- Carson J, *Milk labeling measure debated*, Topeka Capital-Journal, 15 April 2008.

Industry; soft-drink company payments to school districts
- Warner, M. *Lines Are Drawn for Big Suit Over Sodas*, New York Times, 7 December 2005.
- Chmelynski C. *Districts' Vending Machine Contracts Increasingly Under Fire*, School Board News, 12 August 2003.

Ketogenic Diets; clinical uses other than weight reduction
- Wilder RM. *The effects of ketonemia on the course of epilepsy*, Clinical Bulletin *(of the Mayo Clinic)*, Vol 2, p 307 1921.
- Newburgh LH, Marsh PL. *The use of a high fat diet in the treatment of diabetes mellitus*, Archives of Internal Medicine, Vol 26 (6), pp 647-68, 1920.

- Wilder RM, Pollack H. *Ketosis and the ketogenic diet: Their application to treatment of epilepsy and infections of the urinary tract*, International Clinics 1935 pp 1-12, 1935.
- Talbot FB. *Treatment of Epilepsy*, 1 edn. New York: Macmillan; 1930.
- Freeman JM, et al. *The ketogenic diet revisted* In: *Epilepsy Problem Solving in Clinical Practice*, Edited by Schmidt D, Schacter SC. pp 315-324, Martin Dunitz, London, 2000.
- Neal EG, et al. T*he ketogenic diet for the treatment of childhood epilepsy: a randomised controlled trial*, Lancet Neurology, Vol 7 (6), pp 500-6, June 2008

Ketogenic diets; weight reduction, ancient, Hippocratic
- Littré MPÉ: *Du rêgìme â suîvre pour pedre ou gagner de l'embonpoînt*, in: *Oeuvres Complètes D'Hippocrate, traduction nouvelle avec le texte Greg*, vol. 6, pp 76-9, Chez J.B. Baillière, Paris, 1849.

Ketogenic diets; weight reduction, Nineteenth Century
- Banting W. *Letter on Corpulence: Addressed to the Public*, Third Edition, Harrison, London,1864.
- Ebstein W. *Corpulence and Its Treatment on Physiological Principles*, New Edition, H. Grevel & Co.,London,1890 (originally published as *Die Fettleibigkeit (Korpulenz) und ihre Behandung*, Weisbaden, 1882)
- Cohen, IA. *Weight Loss Advice of the Late Nineteenth Century*, American Association for the History of Medicine, Annual Meeting, Birmingham, 2005.
- Cohen, IA. *Nutritional Analysis of Popular Historical Weight-Reduction Diets, Annual Scientific Meeting of the North American Association for the Study of Obesity*, (Abstract Published in Obesity Research, Vol. 13, Page A138, Sept 2005), Vancouver, 2005.
- Cohen, IA: *Analysis of Historic Medical Knowledge Concerning Obesity and Diet*, Prevention 2006-Annual Scientific Meeting of the American College of Preventive Medicine, Reno, 2006.

Mental health; and diet
- Stoll, AL. *The Omega-3 Connection*, Simon & Schuster, New York, 2001.
- Simontacchi C, *The Crazymakers: How the Food Industry is Destroying Our Brains and Harming Our Children*, Tarcher/Putnam, New York, 2000.

Liquid diets; ineffective method
- Tieken SM, et al. *Effects of solid versus liquid meal-replacement products of similar energy content on hunger, satiety, and appetite-regulating hormones in older adults* Hormone Metabolism Research, Vol 39(5) pp389-94, May 2007.

Low-fat dieting; ineffectiveness

- Howard BV, et al. *Low-Fat Dietary Pattern and Weight Change Over 7 Years; The Women's Health Initiative Dietary Modification Trial*, Journal of the American Medical Association, Vol 295, pp 35-49, 2006.
- Shai I, et al *Weight Loss with a Low-Carbohydrate, Mediterranean, or Low-Fat Diet*, New England Journal of Medicine, Vol 359 (3) pp229, 17 July 2008

Life span and diet; ancient
Herodotus, circa 440 BC, recounts a discussion between dignitaries of Ethiopia and Persia, when the Ethiopians criticized the Persian use of bread, stating they would live many more years by avoiding it.
- Rawlinson G (translator),The History of Herodotus, Book III, http://classics.mit.edu/Herodotus/history.3.iii.html (accessed 18 Aug 2008)

Hippocrates circa 400 BC "Those who are naturally of a full habit die suddenly, more frequently than those who are slender."
- Coar T. *The Aphorisms of Hippocrates with a translation into Latin and English*, A.J. Valpy, London, 1822

Life Span and diet; modern
- Masoro EJ *Dietary restriction-induced life extension: a broadly based biological phenomenon*, Biogerontology, Vol 7(3), pp153-5, June 2006.

MSG; hidden
- www.msgmyth.com (accessed 18 Aug 2008).
- Anglesey DI. *Battling the MSG myth*, *A Survival Guide and Cookbook*, Front Porch, Richland, Washington, 2007.

MSG; increased appetite
- Hermanussen M, et al. *Obesity, voracity, and short stature: the impact of glutamate on the regulation of appetite*, European Journal of Clinical Nutrition, Vol 60 (1) pp 25-31, January 2006.
- Hermanussen M, Tresguerres JA. *Does high glutamate intake cause obesity?*, Journal of Pediatric Endocrinology and Metabolism, Vol 16 (7), pp 965-8, September 2003.

MSG; toxicity and health problems
- Schwartz, GR. *In Bad Taste: The MSG Syndrome*, Health Press, Santa Fe 1988.
- Blaylock RL *Excitotoxins: The Taste that Kills*, Health Press, Santa Fe, 1994.

Natural; misuse in food labeling
The best way to understand the misuse of the word "natural" is to read this FDA docket on the red dye made from crushed beetles labeled as a natural product.
- http://www.fda.gov/ohrms/dockets/98fr/E6-1104.htm (accessed 18 Aug 2008).

Obesity epidemic; ancient India
Indian physicians were able to describe an epidemic of obesity and diabetes and identify its cause as sugar consumption more than 1,500 years ago. Recent research has validated the ancient Indian descriptions of Type 2 diabetes.

- Suzarta, as cited by Woodyatt. *Disease of Metabolism* (chapter of A *Textbook of Medicine, Fifth Edition*, Cecil & Kennedy editors) 1941.
- Kar et al. *Prognosis of Prameha on the basis of Insulin level*, Ancient Science of Life, Vol 16 (4), pp 277-83, April 1997.
- Hardy et al. *Ayurvedic Interventions for Diabetes Mellitus: A systematic review*, AHRQ Technology Assessment 41, U.S. Department of Health and Human Services, 2001.

Obesity epidemic; worldwide
Estimated direct and indirect costs of obesity in the United States were $123,000,000,000 in 2001, but this is not just a U.S. problem. Worldwide, the latest estimates of the World Health Organization and the International Obesity Task Force are that 1,700,000,000 people are currently overweight.
- Hossain P, et al. *Obesity and Diabetes in the Developing World – A Growing Challenge*, New England Journal of Medicine, Vol 356 (3), pp 213-5, 18 January 2007.
- Caballero B. *A Nutrition Paradox - Underweight and Obesity in Developing Countries*, New England Journal of Medicine, Vol 352 (15), pp 1514-6, 14 April 2005.

Pharmaceutical industry; profits and public relations
Industry launches public relations efforts to maintain five billion dollars in annual sales of two-cholesterol lowering drugs which cardiologists found ineffective.
- Rubentsein S, Winslow R. *Schering, Merck Defend Their Drugs as Stocks Suffer*, Wall Street Journal, pp B1-2, 11 April 2008.

Pure Food and Drug Act of 1906; reduced addiction
Before 1906, many people, particularly women, were ill and addicted to over-the-counter patent medicines and tonics. These contained a variety of dangerous drugs, but often these were hidden or secret ingredients. The passage of a law that required manufacturers to label these products had a tremendous impact. Although these drugs were not restricted for another eight years, many people who previously had no

idea what they had been consuming stopped once they realized it was their supposed medicine making them ill.
- http://wings.buffalo.edu/aru/preprohibition.htm (accessed 19 Aug 2008).

Salt; benefits of iodized

The World Health Organization is trying to get the non-industrialized and developing nations to set higher standards for iodized salt. Although industrialized nations have been iodizing salt for about eighty years, Switzerland recognized that reduced salt consumption was undoing this benefit. They recently increased the amount of iodine in table salt. They then studied the health of pregnant women and children and documented the benefits.
- World Health Organization. *Recommended Iodine Levels in Salt and Guidelines for Monitoring Their Adequacy and Effectiveness*, WHO/NUT/96.3, World Health Organization, Geneva, 1996.
- Zimmermann MB. *Increasing the iodine concentration in the Swiss iodized salt program markedly Improved iodine status in pregnant women and children: a 5-yr prospective national study*, American Journal of Clinical Nutrition, Vol 82 (2), pp 388-92, August 2005.

Salt; limit restrictions to those with medical needs
- Alderman M. *Dietary Sodium and Cardiovascular Health in Hypertensive Patients: The Case Against Universal Sodium Restriction*, Journal of the American Society of Nephrology Vol 15 (S), pp S47-50, 2004.

264

Index

A

Accept good things happening to you, 122-123, 128

Actigall™, prevents gallstone formation, 45

Activity level, change in, 130; and exercise pattern, 135; to feel better, 123,128

Adults, target audience for this diet, 248

Advocate, health professional as, 248

African Americans, and obesity, 3

Alcohol, avoidance of on this diet, 206, 248-249; carbohydrate, 206; clear out of house, 40, 65

Almond butter, 108

Almonds, 107

Alternative menus in restaurants, 114

America, health costs in, 21

American Association for the History of Medicine, presentation by Dr. Cohen, 12

American Board of Preventive Medicine, 12

American College of Preventive Medicine, presentation by Dr. Cohen, 12

American food processors add MSG, 71-72

American food-supply manipulation, 17-20

American health objectives, 17-18

American Revolution, and sugar consumption, 133

Americans, numbers overweight, 20-21

Amino acids breakdown, 29-30

Amish farm, 69

Amish-raised meat, 100

Anchovies, avoid fermented, 101

Anchovy sauce, fermented, 71

Animals, fattening of, 22

Antibiotic-free meat, 100

Index

Anti-depressants, and overweight people, 205; and weight gain from, 145

Appearance, and weight loss, 21

Appetite reduction with fat burning, 9

Appetite stimulant, 59

Appetite suppression, 242

Appetizers, 115

Aquatic exercises, 250

Arthritis, and overweight, 22

Arthritis Foundation, 250

Artificial foods, and carbohydrates, 22

Artificial sweeteners, 51, 99, 134, 196

Asia, fatness in, 192-193

Asparagus, 95, 168

Asthma, and overweight, 22

Athletes, and sports drinks replace salt, 195

Athletic departments had salt-tablet dispensers, 195

Atkins, Dr. Robert, 10

Atrophy, 50

Avocado, food to stock, 41; grilled recipe, 183

Avoid engineered fats, 64

Avoid faux foods, 64

Avoid flavor enhancers, 64

B

Bacon, 163, 167, 168; cured with sugar, 103; topping, 96

Bacon rinds, unflavored, 108

Bad messages, ignore, 128

Baked goods, clear out of house, 40, 65; and this diet, 191

Balsamic vinegar, 96

Banting, William, 246

Barbecue sauce, avoid commercial, 98; homemade, 165; and meat sauce recipe, 174

Baseline lab tests and retesting, 133

Bathroom scale, 38, 39, 42

Beans, adding back into diet, 141; avoid, 95, 99; clear out of house, 40, 65; not food to stock, 41

Bears and hibernation, 26

Beet sugar, 83

Beets, avoid, 95

Belly fat, 198-199; warning of future medical problems, 198

Beverage, powdered, 106

BGH, 153

Big belly, see Belly fat

Biochemical changes with weight loss, 251-252

Bipolar disorder and diet, 14

Carbohydrate allowance and baked goods, 191

Carbohydrate, 10 grams, 33

Carbohydrate-high diet, 5

Carbohydrate-intake reduction, 129

Carbohydrates, avoid unnecessary, 64; to sugar, 4

Carbon monoxide and red meat, 100

Cardiology research and fasting, 135

Carrots, 96

Cashew butter, 108

Cashews, 107, 163

Cauliflower, 95

CBC, lab test before dieting, 251

Celery, 95; food to stock, 41; okay on calorie-free fast diet, 51

Celiac disease, 134, 141

Center for Science in the Public Interest, and natural color, 69

Cereals, avoid, 149;clear out of house, 40, 65

Chankonabe stew for Sumo wrestlers, 22

Charts of weight loss, 239, 240

Cheese, 105; carry with you on trips, 116; and constipation, 105; food to stock, 41; shredded, 163, 164

Cheese cubes, 164; as snack food, 105

Cheese products, 105

Chef's salad, 115

Chemical preservatives, 67

Chemistry panel (comprehensive), lab test before dieting, 251

Chewing gum (sugar free), okay on calorie-free fast diet, 51

Chicken, 164, 167, 168; with mole sauce, 167

Chicken mole recipe, 175

Chicken stew, 166, 169; recipe, 176-177

Children, and sugar avoidance, 196; and sweets as special treats, 134; and your dieting knowledge, 148

China, and obesity epidemic in, 3, 21, 83

Chinese government, and obesity in, 192-193

Chinese Restaurant Syndrome, 204

Chipotle sauce, 174

Chips contain MSG, 79

Chocolate dessert, 181

Cholesterol, 5; and this diet, 200-202

Cholesterol level and Eskimo diet, 145

Chronic fatigue syndrome, and lack of sodium, 194

Cider vinegar, 96

D

DA, See Department of Agriculture (DA)

Daily log, and meal plans, 161

Dairy products, 104; and butterfat, 64, 66; with fat removed, 192; real, 149

Delicatessen section, 102-103

Denver omelet, 182

Department of Agriculture (DA), responsibility for food safety, 160

Depression, and diet, 145; and hypothyroidism, 194; and overweight, 22

Desert mixes (except sugar-free), food to clear out, 40, 65

Developing countries and sugar, 83

Dextrose, another name for sugar, 85

DHEA, and reduction in belly fat, 198-199

Diabetes, and low-fat diet, 5; and overweight, 22

Diabetics, 249; and this diet, 197-198; medication monitoring, 144

Diary, 203. See also Daily log

Diet, balance, 129; ineffective and hunger, 2; staring phase, 47-61

Diet card, 114

Diet clubs, 125

Diet drugs, 7

"Diet food," makes people hungrier, 20; makes you eat more, 20

Diet soda, 106, 148, 165

Diet tracking, 59

Dietary fat reduction and carbohydrate increase, 17

Dietary fats, diets emphasizing, 11

Dietary trends to protect you, 11

Dieters, and gallbladder disease, 44

Dieting, failures and unwillingness to see physician, 247-248; highly personal act, 199;

infectious, 148; and your physician, 199-200

Diets, cannot work, 1-2; and hunger, 27-28; and metabolic imbalance, 4

Dinner menu, 163-169

Disease control, 130

Disraeli, Benjamin, 207

Doctor, and this diet, 14-15, 35; stay in touch with, 133; talking to, 199-200; and your diet, 199-200

Doughnuts, clear out of house, 40, 65

Dream weight, 124

Dreams can be realistic, 128

Index

Lipid panel, lab test before dieting, 251

Litré, Émile, 241-242, 247

Living with others, and food choice, 63

Lobbying to silence information on BGH, 153

Lobster, 101

Logs of food eaten, 203; daily, 146; sheets for, 209-238

Longevity, and food intake, 136

Long-term loss chart, 240

Look good, you deserve it, 124, 128

Losing weight, meaning of, 121

Low-carbohydrate diets, 10; high in proteins, 30; moderate in protein, 31; recipes from Internet, 162

Low-fat diets, 5; high in carbohydrates, 30; and high-carbohydrate diets, 17-18; ineffective, 245; and profits for food processors, 18, 66; and sugar calories, 66; and this diet, 192

Low-fat foods, clear out of house, 40, 65; high in sugar, 22-23; and this diet, 192

Low-fat salad dressing, 192

Low salt, see Salt, low-salt

Lunch menu, 163-169

Lunches for children, 149

M

Macronutrients, 247

Magic foods, 4, 11

Magnesium, in calcium supplement, 195

Maintaining weight loss, see Leveling off

Maintenance calories, plan, 136

Maintenance diets, 253

Malt vinegar, 96

Maple syrup, clear out of house, 40, 65

Margarine, artificial, 67; clear out of house, 40, 65; hydrogenated fat source, 80-81 Marketplace, and trustworthy food, 207

Marshall Plan, and food shortages, 136

Maturity, and this diet, 248

Mayonnaise (real), 97-98; for fat-centered partial fast, 52; food to stock, 41;

MCT oil, 44, 45

Meal, sides, 113; splitting, 113

Meal plan, and recipes, 161-187; typical day, 56

Meal preparation, 14

Meals, one per day, 243

Mealtimes, rigidity not required, 130

Measuring body fat at home, 38

Recipe Worksheets, 188-190

Recipes with your ingredients, 162

Red dye, 68-69

Refined cane extract, another name for sugar, 85

Religious leaders and fasting, 29

Resetting metabolism by brief fasts, 131

Restaurants online, 118

Rice, clear out of house, 40, 65; and obesity, 192-193

Ridicule against fat people, 122

Roosevelt, Teddy, 77

S

Salad dressing, 96, 116; containing carbohydrates clear out of house, 40, 65;

spice mixtures for, 96

Salad mixes, food to stock, 41

Salads, when eating out, 115

Salmon, 164, 169; canned, 101; cooked or smoked, 166; recipe, 185

Salt, 78; low-salt, 193-194

Salt restrictions, harmful in healthy people, 193-194

Salt-tablet dispensers, 195

Sardines, 101

Saturated fats, 80

Sausage (MSG-free), food to stock, 41, 100

Sausage link, MSG free, 164, 165, 169

Scale. See Bathroom scale

School, food and beverages at, 149-150

School lunches, 149

Scrambled egg, 165, 166, 168

Seafood, 101

Seasoned salts contain MSG, 79

Secretary of health, 154

Seeds, sunflower and pumpkin, 107

Seizure and fasting, 253

Seizure disorder and fat burning, 28-29

Self-blame for not losing weight, 19

Self-esteem, improvement of, 130; of overweight people, 2; and weight loss, 21

Self-image and weight extended to other areas of life, 124

Seltzer water, 106

Separate food items, 39

Serving size, 91, 92

Servings per container, 91

Sesame oil (unrefined), 97, 169, 197; for fat-centered partial fast, 52; food to stock, 41

Set-point myth, 58

Sexual problems, and overweight, 22

Shaker cheese, 105

Shepherds of central Asia, 145

Shopping, 87-109; tips for, 87

Shortening, avoid, 97; clear out of house, 40, 65

Shortest ingredient list, 87

Short-term loss chart, 239

Shredded cheese, 105, 165, 166, 169

Side dishes, 113

Side orders, 114

Sixty-forty-ten daily plan, 33-34, 57

Skim milk, 67; avoid, 192; base for house paint, 104

Skin calipers, 38

Skin problems, and overweight, 22

Sleep apnea, and overweight, 22

Sleeping on a hard surface, 243

Slimmer you, 121-128

Slow metabolism, 2

Snack foods contain MSG, 79

Snack suggestion, 107. 163-169

Snoring, and overweight, 22

Sodas, 106

Sodium, not salt, 78-79

Sodium lack, 78; and chronic fatigue syndrome, 194; and heat intolerance, 194-195

Sodium restriction, 193

Sodium, not salt as problem, 193

Sodium-restricted diets, 78

Soft drink machines at schools, 150

Soft drinks (except for calorie-free), 83; clear out of house, 40, 65

Sorbitol, 94

Soups (except MSG free), food to clear out, 40, 65; canned or powdered and MSG, 149

Sour cream (not low-fat), 41, 66, 105-106; for fat-centered partial fast, 52

South Pacific Island bat, 71

Soy sauce, clear out of house, 40, 65

Soybean oil, avoid, 97

Spaghetti, clear out of house, 40, 65; and MSG, 149

Sparkling water, 106

Special occasions, 139

Spend more for better food, 87

Spice mixes (if containing MSG), food to clear out, 40, 65

Spices (excluding MSG), okay on calorie-free fast diet, 41, 51, 97

Spinach, 95; food to stock, 41

Sports drinks, loaded with sugar, 195; replace salt, 195

Staff members, and weight, 248

Starchy food, clear out of house, 40, 65

Starting to diet, 47-61

Starvation and obesity, 21

State health leadership, handcuffed, 156

Steady fat-burning state, burns stored energy, 9

Steak, 163

Steak sauce, avoid, 98

Stereotypes about fat people, 122

Stevia, 99, 196

Stillman, Dr. Irwin, 10

Strawberry yogurt, 68-69

Stroke, and overweight, 22

Success points, 128

Successful dieting, and confidence in other areas of life, 60

Sucrose, another name for sugar, 85

Sudden death, and overweight, 22

Sugar, alternative names for, 85; and American diet, 133; and artificial sweeteners, 196; clear out of house, 40, 65; diseases from, 83; and glycogen, 28; health risks from, 84; level and fat, 4; as luxury, 82-83; in small amount on label, 92; when eating out, 204; zero calories on label, 84

Sugar addiction, 83-84

Sugar alcohols, 93-94

Sugar substitutes, 84

Sugar-addicted patients, 252

Sugar-based food craving reduced with fat burning, 9

Sugar-free, 82-85; Metamucil, 43; treats and gas, 95

Sugars, avoid all, 87

Sugary syrups, clear out of house, 40, 65

Sumo wrestlers, 22

Sunflower seeds, 107

Supermarket perimeter, avoid processed foods, 89

Support and help of others, 126, 128; See also Overeaters Anonymous (OA); TOPS

Support group, for dieting patients, 125, 251

Surgeon General, 154-155

Surgery for weight loss, 6, 121, 247

Sweetened foods, 143

Sweetener (calorie-free), food to stock, 41

Sweets, taste for diminishes on diet, 84

Syrups for water, sugar free, 106

V

Vacation, and obsessing about diet, 119

Vegetable broth, 78. See also MSG

Vegetable oils, avoid, 66, 82, 97; healthy ones, 197

Vegetable protein, 78

Vegetable-based meat substitutes, avoid, 197

Vegetables, canned, 99; green (fresh or frozen) food to stock, 41

Vegetarians and this diet, 196-197

Victim, and weight loss, 121-122

Vinegar, 96

Vitamin, and fiber supplements, 197; and mineral supplements (sugar-free) okay on calorie-free fast diet, 51

Vitamin D in calcium supplement, 195

W

Waist measurement, 248

Walk, 118

Water, 106-107, 148; okay on calorie-free fast diet, 51

Water fountains, at schools, 150

Water exercise, 123

Weakened food safety enforcement, 151

Web site, 98

Weight, morning compared to evening, 209

Weight gain, 244; on government recommendation to lose weight, 244

Weight history of patient, 250

Weight loss, charting of, 122, 23-240; lose more below goal, 133; stopped or slowed, 202-203; and support group, 140

What works for you, 130

Whipped cream,104; for fat-centered partial fast, 52; food to stock, 41; recipe for, 178; topping, 167

Whitefish infused with MSG, 101

Whitewash from skim milk, 67

Why we are overweight, 17-23

Williamsburg, Virginia, 67

Wine, 206

Wine vinegar, 96

Winners, stick with them, 128

Winning lifestyle, 60

Women, and gallbladder problems, 44

Worcestershire sauce, food to clear out, 40, 65, 99

World Health Organization, world obesity, 21

Worldwide obesity epidemic, 11

Wrinkles, 140

Notes

Notes

Notes

Notes

Notes

Notes